THE POWER OF LOVE

By

Suzanne Woodward Fenders

DEDICATION

This book is dedicated to Nathan
who was willing to share his story.
Also in memory of my mother,
Marjorie Woodward, who always wanted
me to write about Nathan's early years.

WHAT IS VACTERL ASSOCIATION ?

In the medical world babies born with no anal opening and a malformed limb are considered to be possibilities for VACTERL association. In the 1970'S when Nathan was born with this condition, it was called VATER syndrome and was originally thought to affect three or more of the following systems: Vertebrae, Anal, Trachea, Esophagus, and Renal. We weren't given a name for this disease until he was five or six years old, so it was always referred to as birth defects.

This rare disease has been studied as far back as 1839, when babies generally died because doctors were not equipped to care for them.

From Twentieth Century research, cardiac problems and limb defects have been added to the list. The acronym then became VACTERL association. Therefore out of the acronym, VACTERL Nathan had Vertebrae, Anal, Cardiac, Renal, and Limb. And yet most of his childhood he appeared to be perfectly healthy.

Recent studies indicate VACTERL association appears in one of 10,000 to 40,000 newborns. The word association means a series of specific malformations that occur together more often than it would normally happen by chance. The medical profession has never found a specific cause for this rare disease, according to GARD, which stands for the Genetic and Rare Disorders Information Center. GARD also states that the risk for recurrence of VACTERL association in siblings or child is only 1%. There is no evidence that this is either, hereditary, or because of something the mother did or did not do. The doctors always told me it was a virus that attacked the fetus in the womb.

VACTERL association is a lonely disease. It is so rare that we had never met another person that had this particular disease. We travelled in the military all of Nathan's school life and never met a health provider or worker who had ever seen this condition. It was lonely for Nathan because he had no one besides us to give answers to questions, that were seldom asked out loud. Nathan's situation was so different that it was difficult to figure out ways of caring for the skin breakdown which occurred around his colostomy. As he grew we needed to find ways for him to take care of himself. The nurses were wonderful everywhere we went and they tried to come up with solutions and suggestions for his care. It was a learning situation for all of us to handle the everyday problems of hygiene and keeping the skin healthy.

The purpose of this book is to let people who may have to deal with similar situations know they are not alone, and to share how we handled different circumstances as they surfaced. I pray our true story will give encouragement and hope to the reader.

PREFACE

Recently I had a conversation with my forty-four year old son, Nathan, about his early days as a child with a rare disease, VACTERL association. He expressed a desire to know more about the things that had happened to him before "memory". When a child is born with VACTERL association, he needs immediate surgeries. The majority of these happened to Nathan before he was two years old. I was always happy about that, thinking he wouldn't have to deal with those memories. Now that he is an adult with children of his own; he is curious about his own beginnings.

This book is for him. It is also for other families who may be dealing with the struggle of raising a child with birth defects. It is important for them to know they are not alone in their struggles. When Nathan was born with VACTERL association, I'd never heard of it, nor had any of my friends or family. No one was there to ask questions of, and apart from the medical community, I had very little help for his care. A wise friend from my early days as Nathan's mother told me to "take one day at a time and don't worry about tomorrow." I held that thought many times when doctors told me words I didn't want to hear, about negative possibilities for his future. They thought they were preparing me for what could happen but when I looked at my baby; I only saw a beautiful, hopeful and happy life for him. That doesn't mean we didn't have struggles getting there.

This book is also about a military family and their travels from state to state with a child needing much medical attention. Nathan had three siblings, Paul his older brother, Corey his younger brother and Emily who was ten years younger than him. With a dad often out to sea leaving this young family behind, there were many difficulties that our faith helped us through.

My goal is to be honest and encouraging in this book. Many details I cannot recall at this time in my life, yet there are also so many, still embedded in my memory that I shall never forget. They are the ones the reader will hear about in these pages.

They are the memories of a mother who never wanted to be a nurse because of her repulsion to the sight of blood. Yet one who was able to face greater challenges than she ever could have imagined. When it was necessary, when it was her own baby, it was time to put her own fears aside. "God gives us just enough grace for the step we're on," the saying goes. And with His Grace, this child grew up to be a strong, intelligent, happy contributor to society; and an awesome Dad!

CONTENTS

CHAPTER ONE

SEPTEMBER 6, 1973

Waking up in pain once more, my body wouldn't allow me to forget I'd just given birth. The discomfort of hemorrhaging could in no way equal the pain of separation from my newborn. He was my second son, Nathan, but he wasn't in my arms. Instead, Dr. Brownlow, who had delivered him five hours earlier, was standing by my bed telling me he needed to call my husband home from a Navy deployment to the Vietnam War. Dr. Brownlow was in the Navy Reserves and knew how to get Hank home.

Nathan was born on September 6, 1973 at Blue Hill Memorial Hospital in Blue Hill, Maine. He was 9 pounds, 11 ounces, pink and very healthy looking. In spite of this, he was born with no anal opening. I didn't want to think Nathan's problem was that serious, but the doctor told me he needed surgery within twenty four hours, and the nearest hospital that could do this was three hours away. My mind was filled with worry and bewilderment. There wasn't much explanation for Nathan's condition but I could see the concern in my doctors eyes. My heart ached to be with my baby and hold him but the doctor said it was better for both of us this way.

The overwhelming sadness I was feeling, as well as the weakness in my body, left me with no strength to object.

My body had given birth without the help of any pain killers. It carried an extra bag of water throughout the pregnancy that nobody seemed to detect before it splashed out on the doctor, just after he delivered Nathan. It planned to nurse this baby but now the baby was too far away so there was discomfort and confusion for this body and mind. After a few days of rest, surgery, and a couple pints of blood my body felt almost normal again, but my heart was still aching to be with my newborn once more!

Dr. Brownlow was a next-door neighbor to my parents. He had four children of his own whom I used to babysit before I was married. I trusted him, and he showed a lot of compassion for me and my family. If he wanted to bring Hank home he knew more than I did about Nathan's condition.

But our family's story starts earlier.

CHAPTER TWO

THE UNKNOWN

We cannot always plan our own destiny, although some of us like to try. No matter how many plans we make there's always the possibility that something will happen to change events. Somehow I always thought I'd grow up, get married and have a family, in or near Blue Hill, my home town in Maine. All my family was in this area: my parents, three brothers, many cousins, aunts, and uncles. My mother came from a family of ten children and most of them were right here in Hancock County.

I met my husband, Hank while in college, and we always felt we would be married. But after four years of preparing to be a music teacher; what I wanted to do was teach and live on my own to work and support myself. I wanted to see what it felt like to earn my own paycheck and make my own decisions. I learned good lessons during those two years of teaching: the majority of my check went for rent, electricity, heat, food; but my roommate, Miff and I managed to save enough of our checks to have some fun on weekends.

Miff attended the same college I did. We were both in the music program but she graduated a year before me. She had found a job in a school system that covered three towns and the district really needed another music teacher. Miff was a wonderful friend and asset for me to have as a roommate. She knew the "ropes" of the system as well as the area for shopping, going out to eat, and so on. We rented a third-floor attic apartment with three rooms, a bathroom and an unfinished storage room. A Rope ladder was placed near the kitchen window at my Dad's insistence, because there was only one entrance to the apartment

Hank would come and visit and stay in a spare room downstairs in an old lady's apartment. He was very patient and promised to wait for me to be ready to get married.

The shock came when I went to graduate school in Potsdam, New York - the summer after college graduation and returned to find Hank had joined the Navy! Hank's plans were very contrary to my intentions. Now what? That didn't fit my plan book. I never said I wanted to be a Navy wife! I would have to wait for him to complete boot camp and receive leave time to come home to be married. So, you see someone had to change her attitude and make up her mind what was important.

*   *   *

May 17, 1970 at two p.m., I was standing in the vestibule of the Blue Hill Baptist Church, staring towards the front of the church. The church was full of family and friends and the day was cloudy and showery and it just didn't feel real for some reason. Hank was so tall and handsome, standing there waiting for me. Music began to play, and our family doctor, Dr. Brownlow, who would later deliver my second son Nathan, and his wife, Jackie was singing from the balcony with the organ. They had beautiful voices that sounded amazing with the organ, and I was happy they could be there that day.

There were bridesmaids in pastel dresses, carrying baskets of pastel colored flowers in front of me. As they proceeded down the aisle, I followed behind my best friend's three-year old daughter, who tossed rose petals as she walked. Jenny was an adorable blue-eyed, blonde flower girl. When I arrived on the arm of my Dad, to face my soon - to - be husband, I thought my heart would jump out of my chest! My mind was racing: what were we thinking?

We hardly knew each other.   Well, it had been two years since we met.   But our whole relationship had been based on letters and phone calls with an occasional date if we happened to be in the same state!   We knew so little about each other. Yet we loved each other, and here we were.   He was so attractive and calm looking, while inside I felt the whole event seemed surreal.   I willingly walked into a totally unfamiliar world and couldn't even imagine what lay ahead for us; but felt compelled to take this step with this calm, in control, person. Hank was exactly what I needed.

Hank had arrived from Florida the day before and I told him we needed to memorize our vows. It just seemed more authentic to me. If you plan to be married for a lifetime, you should mean your vows enough to memorize them; at least that was my way of thinking. So he agreed and worked hard to do just that the night before the wedding.

There we were: Hank was holding my hands saying his vows with no hesitation, and when it was my turn my mind went blank. The pastor said the first couple words to help me start the sentence and then realized my brain was totally paralyzed! He fed me every phrase of my vows; I was so nervous I could barely talk. My heart was pounding, my mouth was dry, and I couldn't understand where all these nerves were coming from.

After the pastor said "You may kiss the bride", and Hank kissed me; there was a feeling that everything was right and whatever the unknowns were in the future we could face together. I totally relaxed and shed all of my concerns. Someone started to giggle and the pastor touched our shoulders to announce "Mr. and Mrs."   Little did we know what the future would hold for us as we set out on this road together.

CHAPTER THREE

STARTING A FAMILY

From our wedding we headed to Key West, Florida where Hank was still stationed. A new adventure of marriage and travel lay before us. After one month that felt like a honeymoon for me, although Hank had to work, he was sent to Bremerton, Washington to board a Navy Destroyer Escort headed for Hawaii. The *USS Whipple* would be his ship and home away from home for the next three years. I reluctantly went back to Blue Hill and stayed with my parents that summer where I found a job waitressing at the local restaurant. It would have been too costly for me to try to travel with Hank at this time. He would have to settle in Hawaii and then find housing for us before I could join him. So military life had started for us; married and together one month; separated for four months.

The waitress job was fun because I met other waitresses who knew how to enjoy themselves while doing hard work. It helped me keep my weight down as I was in motion all the time. Blue Hill is a summer tourist town and I loved meeting new people. Sometimes visitors to our town would sail into the harbor and come to the restaurant for a special meal. The days seemed to pass quite quickly because the job kept me so busy and tired. I expected a call any day that would be my trip to Hawaii, to bring me back to my husband once again. That call didn't come by the end of the summer when the restaurant business slowed down at the end of the tourist season, and most of the waitresses were let go. So it was time to look for a new job.

A superintendent in the area was looking for a substitute music teacher. His music teacher had hurt her back moving a piano (a common problem of music teachers, I learned). I applied for the job, making sure he understood my dilemma and that I would leave as soon as my husband called. He liked to tease me and say Hank would take his time to enjoy Hawaii and the hula girls there before he called for me to join him. I assured him Hank wasn't like that and we both wanted to be reunited as soon as possible. Still he would tease me and seemed to have all kinds of confidence that I would be there all fall, if not the whole semester! Teaching was very rewarding and enjoyable but at this time my heart and mind were in faraway places.

The call came from the airport one afternoon in October during school hours. My mother took the message that my ticket to Hawaii had been paid for and was waiting at the airport for me to pick up the next day at eight am. With less than twelve hours to do laundry, pack my clothes, pack a few wedding gifts, we might be able to use in our apartment in Hawaii, and say some quick good – byes, I was ready to depart early in the morning. I never saw my friend, the superintendent again.

Boarding the plane I was filled with a great anticipation of the future. Flying into this vast unknown was very exciting but still a frightening experience for me. There was so much to learn about military life. But for now I could hardly wait to see my husband! Our new venture together had begun. Hank was right there waiting when the plane arrived after my twelve hour flight. I was so overjoyed to finally see him again after such a long separation. My heart said "Now I'm home, we're finally together!"

We had a two bedroom apartment in Navy leased housing in downtown Honolulu. Our apartment was on the third floor, with no elevator. We didn't mind because we were young and just happy to be together. After settling in and getting to know my surroundings a little, I decided to start looking for a job. Naturally the first place to start would be the public schools. However, the public school jobs were almost always taken by the island people. Other avenues would have to be pursued.

Meanwhile, Hank and I had an opportunity to go on a weekend cruise on his ship to Maui. We enjoyed exploring another island for a while. It also gave family members a taste of what life on the USS Whipple was like.

It was the end of October when I arrived in Honolulu, so I went to some of the larger stores to apply for a holiday job. They were looking for someone to wrap packages for the Christmas season. It was a relaxing job, consisting of basically putting ribbons on pretty boxes. When Christmas was over my search for another job began.

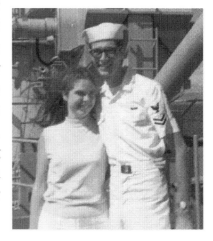

A neighbor, Maxine, told me about a preschool looking for a teacher. She worked at the one located at an Episcopal Church, nearby. It sounded like a fun job so I decided to apply and was accepted. My responsibility was to create a music program and run a class of seventeen four year olds at the same time. I fell in love with the little Hawaiian children and it turned out to be a great job for me. Those were warm happy days. I certainly received an education on what raising small children would be like. Hank and I began to think of starting our own family.

The preschool job lasted about nine months for me. By then I was seven months pregnant with my first child. That summer the weather was very hot so in the afternoon I would stop and buy a snow cone before boarding the bus home after work, craving watermelon sherbet. We found a place in Waikiki that we liked to go on weekends that made watermelon sherbet, so we frequented that area as well. To this day my now 45 year old son, Paul loves watermelon sherbet.

Paul was born in December of 1971 and we decided to name him after both of our fathers, Paul Henry. Our new baby was our pride and joy. Both of us missed our families, and dreamed of taking him to visit grandparents and show him off, but they were just too far away. For now we would enjoy him ourselves, knowing that one day in the future he would meet his grandparents. Paul loved the zoo and when he was old enough we took him there often. Beach days were his favorite. When he was little Hank would build a little pool right at the waters' edge for him to sit in. The sand would give Paul support around his back. At our apartment building there was a small pool where we sometimes took him swimming. By the age of nine months he was old enough to be enrolled at the local YWCA for swim lessons. Paul would swim under water and come up smiling every time. We could almost tell at that time he would always love the water and swimming.

Nine weeks after Paul was born Hank's ship went on a WESTPAC deployment(Vietnam) . The USS Whipple left with a fleet of five ships out of Pearl Harbor and we knew we shouldn't expect to see them for seven months. After saying goodbye to my husband, I took my tiny son and drove back to our quiet, empty apartment, with tears in my eyes most of the way. It was definitely a desolate and empty feeling returning to that apartment knowing Hank wouldn't be coming home for months. Never before had I felt so alone as that first long separation from him. There were a few people around the apartment complex that I knew a bit and I decided this would be the time to make some new friends. I knew there would be no point in a pity party so it was time to plan a routine for Paul and me. Also, there were projects, such as rug hooking, I had planned to keep myself busy.

Being in Hawaii during the Vietnam War, we received news on TV that was a little different than the mainland news. I always watched the eleven pm news before going to bed. Occasionally I could actually see our ships. One night the news said one of our ships, in the fleet of five, was hit. Naturally all the wives were very nervous about this. The captain's wife was busy calling all the ship's wives and finally did call me. She said Hank's ship was the one hit but the damage wasn't too serious and no one was hurt. Between seeing the news and finally getting the call from our captain's wife, was a terribly stressful time for all of the waiting families.

I allowed myself one phone call a week to my mother in Maine. There were no cell phones then and long distance calls were extremely expensive. My friend Maxine, who lived at the other end of my floor, was moving as her husband was being stationed somewhere on the mainland. The two of us had become good friends working at the preschool together, and I would dearly miss her.

When Paul was four months old, my Mom flew to Hawaii to visit for one short week. She came with a tour group and stayed with me and Paul. My Mom was always my best friend and I had missed her terribly. We had so much to talk about and I loved the time we spent with her that week. She wanted to spend time rocking and singing to her grandson and he was always willing to have her. We decided to go to the mall and have pictures taken of Paul. I realized then that Hank was never going to see his son at this age.

Paul was nine months old when Hank finally came home. All the wives and families were on the pier at Pearl Harbor with the brass bands and hula girls. What an extraordinary celebration! The feeling of excitement and community being on that pier will always stay with me. Everyone there was feeling the same expectations of seeing a loved one who had been gone for months. The day turned out to be like Christmas because Hank had saved all his money to buy things in the Philippine Exchange, that were so much cheaper there than they were here. It was exciting to see all he had brought us but even more fun for him to see his son, and to have Paul see his Dad!

Arriving at the apartment, Paul was put on the floor where he crawled everywhere. He drooled profusely as he was crawling! At first Hank set out to clean the floor wherever Paul had drooled. He ran to get a paper towel for every puddle and I sat there and laughed. The two of them were extremely entertaining to watch! We had many happy days in Hawaii and a few very stressful ones, like the night Hank was called back to the ship in the middle of the night. There was no reason given on the phone or even an explanation of when he'd be home. I didn't hear from him for two weeks, a worrisome situation for all the wives. We called the captain's wife but even she had no information to give us. When the men came home we learned they were out chasing unauthorized Russian submarines coming down from Alaska that were too close to the Hawaiian Islands.

Our lives had become tentative; we had no idea when Hank would come or go or be transferred somewhere else. We did know in the late spring of 1973 that Hank would be deployed once again on a Westpac in the Vietnam waters. I was pregnant with our second child and this time we decided I should take Paul and go to my parents' home in Blue Hill to have the baby. There would be a lot of help with Paul from my parents, and my Mom and Dad were just aching to see their young grandson. At this time Paul was about sixteen months and a big helper for me. After we saw Hank's ship off for his second deployment to Vietnam, Paul and I started packing. Well, I was packing and he was mostly unpacking. He thought it was a game but it was exhausting for me because I was trying to defrost a refrigerator at the same time. Every time I went back to put more things in the suitcase, he had taken the contents out and thrown them on the floor. We played this game until I finally gave up and waited for his naptime to finish packing.

Paul was happy to be going somewhere but he certainly didn't understand what the day would be like or the exciting adventure he would have on his first airplane flight. Ann, my neighbor and friend, offered to take us to the airport. We were both about seven months pregnant and dragging a large suitcase down three flights to the parking garage under our apartment building, along with a toddler to help down. If you ever notice in a large store or mall when a woman with small children is having trouble with doors, it's usually another woman or pregnant woman who will assist her. I was truly thankful for my friend Ann that day.

The flight was endlessly long and tiring for both of us. We had seats in the front of a 747, near the stewardess' station. She was good to me and put me there so Paul would have floor space to play on if he wanted to. Not a chance! Neither playing nor a nap was on Paul's radar. He was there to explore. So the stewardess said, "Just let him go, he's not going anywhere." She offered to watch him while I took a nap; I obviously looked like I needed it more than he did. Paul ran up front around the bar area and someone suggested giving him a drink to slow him down! I decided to take the stewardess' advice and after a few minutes someone from the back of the plane came up carrying a crying baby boy.

When we arrived in Bangor, Maine, my Mom was there to meet us and she hardly recognized me; I was completely exhausted with no chance for sleep for that whole twelve hour trip. I was looking forward to the stop in San Francisco so we could get off the plane and stretch our legs. But that turned out to be the only part of the trip that Paul fell asleep! Everyone else got off the plane and there we sat; Paul sound asleep on my lap.

Paul and I were very excited to be in Maine with my parents. At the same time we were both so tired from the long trip we needed a nap before dinner. Up until now he had slept in a crib. Mom didn't have one so we put him in a twin bed in the room right next to me. Paul received so much love and attention from his grandparents, he became very comfortable in Blue Hill and very happy to be there. I also appreciated their company and being able to share the responsibility of this little guy.

We spent the summer with my parents waiting for Nathan's arrival. My mother had an office just off her living room, where she did bookkeeping for a couple doctors. When she was working, I kept Paul busy somewhere else. Later she would take coffee breaks and we would watch the happenings of the Watergate trials. 1973 was the summer of Watergate! I spent a lot of that summer with my swollen ankles up on a hassock, watching the trial on TV .

It was a long summer with little communication from Hank because of his deployment, and the fact there was no modern technology. As time came closer to the birth I began to look forward with great anticipation to having this second child and taking him or her back to Hawaii to see their Dad. Sometimes our best plans just don't turn out the way we anticipate. I never did go back to Hawaii.

CHAPTER FOUR

NATHAN

At the end of the summer I was huge and dreadfully uncomfortable. I had to sit with my feet up because of swelling in my legs and my labor started early, causing more discomfort. There was such a feeling of discouragement when they sent me home from the hospital because labor stopped. Relief came when I finally gave birth to a beautiful , healthy-looking nine pound, eleven ounce baby boy! When Nathan was born the nurse tried to take his temperature and discovered he had no anal opening. She also noticed an extra thumb on his right hand that seemed to come out of the base of this main thumb. These were the first two indications that anything was wrong.

Dr. Brownlow came in to tell me what they had found or, rather, not found on my baby. He explained that during in utero development, every opening in the body dimples out and dimples in until it meets and makes an opening. He said my baby's colon could be just behind the skin and then it would only be necessary to cut the skin away. The other alternative was that the colon may not have developed enough to come all the way down.

In that case, he would need major, lifesaving surgery which would result in a colostomy on his abdomen. My immediate response was that I was very sure it would just be a matter of cutting the skin away and everything would be fine. Paul had been so healthy, and by all accounts, other than an extra thumb, Nathan looked to be very healthy as well. That's all it was, Dr. Brownlow would see. So I fell asleep confident that he would find out I was right.

After further examination later that morning, Dr. Brownlow came back to tell me Nathan needed to be sent to Maine Medical Center in Portland. It had been arranged that my mother and aunt, who was a nurse, would take him. He said I would be allowed to hold Nathan once before they left. In my mind these words were unacceptable and I wanted to argue with him that there must be some mistake! I still couldn't fathom the fact Nathan wasn't healthy. My heart began to feel deprived of my beautiful baby boy. Being allowed to hold him only once seemed so unreal to me and I started missing him the minute they took him away. My only consolation was knowing he was in good hands with my Mom and Aunt Muriel, which gave me a lot of peace. They would be very careful with the precious cargo they needed to deliver to the medical center in Portland.

Nathan arrived with his grandmother and great aunt, Dr. Bell, the pediatric surgeon expecting them, immediately took him into surgery. It was necessary to put a colostomy in his abdomen so his colon could empty. These things were explained to me but I was only twenty seven and very inexperienced as far as medical terms were concerned. I couldn't grasp what my poor baby was going through in a hospital three hours away. All I could think of was getting better so I could go see him.

Nathan was born with VACTERL association, a term I had never heard before, and I had no idea what lay ahead for my baby to endure.

Nathan's Dad was in the South Vietnam waters, on his second Westpac trip, when he got the message from the Red Cross to come home as soon as possible. The message was brief and sent to the Captain of the ship. Hank had no more information about the baby or me – as communication on ships in the 1970's was not as good as it is today. So Hank set out on a week long journey with no understanding of the baby's condition.

The Red Cross message from Dr. Brownlow arrived when Hank's ship was in the Gulf of Tonkin, Vietnam. The ship pulled into Singapore, where he was given a ride to the Air Force base. He flew on an Air Force cargo plane, sitting on a cargo net flying sideways. After arriving in the Philippines Hank had a two day wait before boarding the Flying Tiger Airlines, a military commercial chartered plane. On this flight the altimeter was not working and the plane was forced to land in Japan. Hours were spent in that airport waiting for the parts to arrive. Following the repair of the altimeter they flew on to Anchorage, Alaska. Hank said it was the first time he'd flown into a sunrise.

The next stop after Anchorage was Traverse Air Force Base in California. A commercial flight had been held up waiting for Hank. If a serviceman is travelling on an emergency leave the airlines try to accommodate them. He was very thankful for that.

Hank had been wearing the same set of dress whites since he left the ship several days earlier. The commercial flight was a welcomed and much appreciated relief from the cargo planes, giving him an opportunity to change clothes. Two more stops and he would be in Maine.

Making this long trip home alone with his thoughts, Hank couldn't even imagine that Nathan's problem would be so serious. He was thinking as I did, that our first child, Paul was so healthy, Nathan's condition wouldn't be terribly complicated. We both were wrong on that count.

I had been sent back to the Blue Hill Hospital a week after giving birth, with problems of my own from child-birth, even as Nathan was still in the Portland hospital. The day Hank arrived home I was being discharged from the hospital and he picked me up. We were so happy and relieved to see each other after months of separation and all the trials we each endured on our own. There would be so much to catch up on, but for now our complete focus was Nathan. After I explained everything that had happened to Nathan, Hank talked to Dr. Brownlow. He told Hank the basic information and attempted to give us encouragement by saying, "If you treat Nathan normal, he will be normal." I've always remembered those words which became an important part of our parenting. Nathan received the same treatment as his siblings. He was given the same disciplines, hugs, chores, and rewards as the others. He definitely grew up normally, even as he was compelled to survive in a not so normal body.

It was two weeks after Nathan's birth when the call came from Dr. Bell. Nathan was ready to come home! I had been so worried about him and it felt like the nurses knew my son better than his own mother. Whenever I called, they always assured me he was a wonderful patient. He had a good disposition and they all favored him, and kept him at the nurses' station often. They tried to give him extra attention because we weren't able to be there.

We were already to set out for Portland when the first phone call, of what would be many, stopped us. Nathan's ureters had backed up urine into his kidney and the doctors needed to immediately take care of that. It meant Nathan would need surgery again right away. Dr. Bell asked us to wait a few days longer so he could observe that the surgery was successful. It seemed like an eternity before we could finally go see him.

Nathan was nearly three weeks old before his father saw him for the first time. When the day finally came for us to make the trip to Portland, the whole family was excited. Paul would spend the day with his grandparents while Mom and Dad would bring his baby brother home.

Upon arrival at the hospital we met Nathan's doctor. Dr. Bell had us come to his office before we saw our baby. He explained that Nathan now had a colostomy and two ureterostomies on his abdomen. The ureterostomies were parts of the ureter pulled to the side of his abdomen. The urine would drain through them until, at some later date to be chosen, the doctor would close them. While he was talking I kept thinking, "How can I do this? I'm not a nurse!" But the overwhelming love I felt for this child kept me from thinking anything but "We can do this." Dr. Bell was a kind, gentle, and honest man and he wanted us to know that Nathan's surgeries were not over. He told us there would be a "series" of them. I couldn't hear this and Hank didn't want to either. We just wanted to take our child home and love him into being healthy. Dr. Bell must have been able to see the fear in our faces as he was talking. We wanted to know specifics but he wisely had nothing to tell us. He said each child was different so we would have to take it one day at a time.

We explained to the doctor how Hank had signed up in the Navy for six years and then was planning to get out. (Our plan was a home in Blue Hill near my family.) Dr. Bell was so kind to us saying, "Don't change your plans. You can pay me according to what you can afford, and I think the hospital will say the same." To say the least, we were shocked that he would say that to us! But while we appreciated his compassion for our situation, neither of us could do that. It was never a question of what we'd do. The military was the best place for us to be so Nathan would get the best care.

Dr. Bell had some good advice to give us as we began this frightening journey of being Nathan's parents. He instructed us to always speak to the doctor in charge whenever we took Nathan to the hospital. That statement alone indicated there would be more trips to the hospital, and added to our nervousness. However it was good advice and we always made sure to do that. Our choice to stay in the military turned out to be the best, because one year later Dr. Bell transferred to a hospital in Missouri.

The moment had finally come when we could go see our baby together. Dr. Bell sent us to the nurses at the neo-natal ward for them to show us how to care for Nathan. When we arrived he was all swaddled in the little crib and looked so peaceful. We held him and talked to him. He seemed to respond to us right away and it felt like he was finally where he belonged: in our arms. Then it was time to learn how to diaper him. When the nurse took Nathan's diaper off, I heard my mind saying "God help me, I can't do this! I can't do this!!" With Hank's jet-lag from all the time zones he'd recently travelled through, he became very light headed and the nurse quickly gave him a chair. Hank had never before or since fainted for any reason.

Our first reaction was a surreal feeling of being totally overwhelmed, unable to imagine how we'd take care of this child. Of course, neither could we imagine not taking care of him. Initially I wanted to cry: my mind was racing! How could I do this? Which nurse can I take home with me?? But I pulled myself together and told myself, " We can do this. Whatever we have to do, we will. He is our baby and there's no alternative. We love this little guy so much we will work together and care for him." All these thoughts were tumbling around in my mind at once!

The nurse was compassionate and kind. Step by step, she showed me how to put the creams and dressings on my baby's three openings on his abdomen, for the colostomy and two ureterostomies. The diaper then wrapped around his belly leaving his little bottom without coverage. There was no need. He then was swaddled in blankets and passed to me to take home. The nurses wrote instructions for the diaper change and I prayed this wouldn't have to be done before we arrived at my parents' home. With the support of my mother, I would be able to learn this routine. No matter what had to be done for our baby, he would get the best care we could give.

Blue Hill is a small community and news travels fast. Having grown up in this town I knew everyone probably had heard about Nathan's situation. I was sure the Baptist Church my family attended would be praying for him. It gave me a lot of peace knowing there were people praying for my baby.

The drive home was long and quiet. We hardly knew what to say. This whole situation was more than anything either of us had ever had to handle. We knew this wouldn't be easy for us but couldn't possibly understand what would lie ahead for our Nathan and our family.

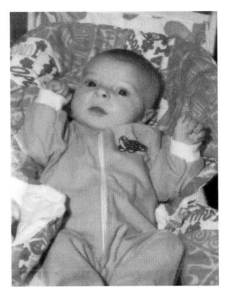

CHAPTER FIVE

THE ANGEL NEXT DOOR

There was a new sound in the Woodward House on Parker Point Road in Blue Hill! Suddenly a parade of grandmother, mother, big brother and dog were all racing towards this sound: a baby crying!

Hank and I had arrived late the night before with Nathan; too late to introduce him to his big brother, Paul. It was morning and Nathan was hungry, so I fixed his bottle and was disappointed at how little he would actually take of it. Now grandparents and brother wanted a turn to hold him. Nathan responded right away to Paul, who was very curious about this new "person of interest" in his realm. He had pretty much won the apple of Grandma's eye award already. But this little guy was fascinating to him and Mom would need his help to change the diaper.

Paul had collected a couple of his special toys to show his new baby brother. Things just seemed to go more smoothly if he kept the baby's interest while I changed the diaper. Immediately when the diaper came off, the stoma, or opening of the colostomy, needed attention. First, all gauze pads had to be thrown away, and the cloth diaper went into the diaper pail. Nathan's abdomen was washed with warm, soapy water and then dried completely. The nurses had made a cream mixture of brewer's yeast, Desitin, and karaya gum powder to go around the stoma to heal and protect the skin. Once that was on, a pile of gauze pads covered the opening. The ureterostomies were treated similarly with a softer cream and then gauze pads. The diaper was then folded in thirds the long way and wrapped around his abdomen, pinned snuggly. Next, he was dressed in a zip-up sleeper and wrapped in a blanket.

Now, finally the time had come when Paul could hold his brother. What a picture! Nathan has a smile on his face as if he were ready to play. Paul looks so sweet and just happy to have his little brother home. The picture showed Nathan's extra thumb, which would one day be removed - but not soon enough for Mom. It seemed to catch up on his clothing easily, and I kept asking with each surgery: "Can't you just take that off at the same time?" The answer was always, "We will , but this little guy has enough complications to go through right now."

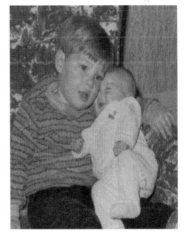

My parents' support was crucial at this time. Whenever I got discouraged, Dad would reassure me that Nathan would be fine. Mom kept reminding me that I could handle this. She showed me courage when I faltered and stayed affirming and upbeat around me. I secretly knew her heart was breaking for all this baby was going through but we both kept a stiff upper lip. The special care of Nathan was so new to us, we had to put him before our emotions. Life was intense for a while.

Hank had to go back to Hawaii to pack up our belongings and clean the apartment. Before he went, he and I took a day to go visit the chaplain at the Brunswick Air Station. The chaplain explained that the hospital in Hawaii would not be able to handle Nathan's needs, so Hank would need an immediate transfer. Since we had family in Maine and Massachusetts he should be transferred somewhere in New England, close to hospitals that could help Nathan. The Navy was giving Hank a transfer to Groton, Connecticut, where these hospitals could be easily accessed. At first I didn't understand why we couldn't take Nathan back to Hawaii with us. There's a huge Army hospital there on the island but Nathan's doctors decided for us, that he should be here, in New England, where there were plenty of doctors, and our families. Family support is very important for anyone going through a catastrophic illness. The professionals knew we would be needing specialists for future surgeries as well.

Two weeks had passed since Hank arrived in Blue Hill and now it was time for him to go. The boys and I would stay with my parents until he had made arrangements for us to move. Hank was sent back to Hawaii where he would be stationed, temporarily, on a submarine tender because his ship was still in Vietnam. While he was in Hawaii Hank had to work every day, come home to the empty apartment to pack up our belongings, and then ship them to my parents' home in Blue Hill. After packing and clearing everything out, he had to clean the apartment for the next renters.

A few phone calls from Hank at the pay phone booth at the Ala Moana Shopping Mall in Waikiki made me homesick for the life we'd had for the last two and a half years in Hawaii. I could hear through the phone the sounds of people enjoying themselves and even Hank sounded happier. In spite of the ordeal our family was going through, he must have found Hawaii to be quite a contrast to life in Blue Hill, maybe even a welcome relief. My friend Ann, who had helped

Paul and me get to the airport, was pregnant. She was due any day, and her sister had come to be with her during this time because Ann's husband was on the ship Hank had just left. Hank let her know he was around if she needed any help. He told me of things he did to help Ann and he even went out to eat with them.

I loved my husband and knew he loved me, but I began to feel emotionally insecure. I know it was hormones but my imagination was not my friend at this time. My days and nights were long and hard and I began to feel jealous of him, not even realizing what an ordeal he was actually going through himself, at work and making preparations to return. He was able to drive around Hawaii, see our friends, feel the warm breezes on his face. Although I loved my boys and couldn't bear to be away from them, some days I found myself fighting tears all day. With very little communication from my husband it made me wonder what the future would be: if he would still be there for us. Realizing my feelings of insecurity, one day my mother said, "There's a nurse named Carol who lives next door. Would you like me to call her and see if she'd come over?" My response was a very enthusiastic "YES!"

Carol was a Mom of three children and recently had decided to give up her job to be at home with them. She was so cheerful and always had a smile and a positive word of encouragement. She was also very smart in the nursing field and seemed to know just what we needed to do for Nathan. After all, when I got discouraged about Nathan's personal care, I would call a doctor and they'd tell me to ask the nurses. Carol was a gift to be living right next door! If Carol didn't know an answer, she'd always find out or make a suggestion where to look for one. I found myself calling her often for advice.

Between Carol, my mother, and myself we were able to come up with ways to be more efficient with the diaper change. For example we took Chux pads and cut pieces to go over the gauze on Nathan's stoma to prevent leakage through his clothes. Since Carol was a nurse and had to be creative at her job, her suggestions and medical expertise proved so valuable to us!

Soon Carol was coming over every morning after she got her kids off to school. She had a wonderful way about her that seemed to help me feel more confident in my care of my son. Carol kept looking and commenting on what we were doing that worked well. And then she would add suggestions for things that might improve our situation. I really began to depend on her daily visit as she became a particularly vital friend during these days. One of the best things about Carol was her attitude of positivity towards Nathan and his care. She helped me feel almost "normal" about his daily routine care that had to be done. So, a new normal in baby care. Carol had a wonderful sense of humor and I can remember her laughing over one thing or another. With kids, there's always something to find humor in, especially with a two - year - old toddler named Paul, around.

The fall after Nathan was born was a very nice extension of summer days. My mother bought us a carriage for Nathan, and I would put him in it for a nap in the warm September sun. Our family has always been a big fan of fresh air and believe every child should be out in the sunshine daily. So I started my children young, taking them for rides or allowing them to nap outside if it was warm. If Nathan was in the carriage napping, my mother's dog, Scampy, was right beside the carriage. He was extremely protective of my children. He'd lie down and sleep on the ground and growl if anyone came near.

One time we couldn't find Paul. Carol had come over for her daily visit so she helped us look. Carol, Dad, Mom and I looked everywhere, inside and outside of the house. Mom noticed Scampy wasn't around so she said "Paul's alright, Scamp must be with him." My Aunt Anna lived down the road from my parents and I'd taken Paul to see her often so we decided to check there. Carol offered to stay with Nathan while the rest of us went to see Aunt Anna. Paul had found his way down the sidewalk, under the barn at Anna's house and, Mom was right, Scampy sat close beside him. Both of them seemed very happy and content together, surprised that we were all there looking for them. We wondered if Paul had followed Scampy under the building, or if it was vice versa.

One morning Carol came over for her usual visit. I was upset because Nathan was very pale and his lips were blue. It scared me but she said to check his fingernails. If they were blue as well, then it could indicate a heart problem. Thankfully, the nails were still pink. Nathan was also refusing to eat and that worried me, so I did call the doctor. He assured me all babies like to eat and I should just be patient. It turned out there was more wrong than just not eating well. The next morning Nathan woke up with labored breathing and projectile vomiting. It frightened me so much I immediately called Carol, who said, "Call the doctor NOW". The doctor was my family doctor, Dr. Brownlow, who had delivered Nathan, as we didn't have a pediatrician in Blue Hill at this time. After Dr. Brownlow examined Nathan, he wasn't sure if it was bronchitis, so he called a pediatrician at the hospital in the next town. When he got off the phone he looked at me and said, "If he were my child I'd take him to Portland." And so we did. The beginnings of bronchitis was what the doctors decided was the problem. It was one of many times Nathan would spend a week in the hospital getting healthy again.

Nathan was in the hospital. Hank was in Hawaii. Mom was in her office trying to work. Paul and I were just waiting to hear some good news from somebody. I always felt so helpless when Nathan was hospitalized because I couldn't take care of him. These were emotional times for me. My thoughts went between worrying about him and how they would get him better, and did I fail to keep him well? It was stressful for me when doctors showed their insecurities concerning his care. Dr. Brownlow was not the only one. Many times, when taking Nathan to dispensaries on the military bases, I would get a doctor or physician's assistant that seemed to have no idea what to do with this child. In those cases, we usually took him right to Children's Hospital in Boston. They always handled things as if they'd done the same thing many times, which I'm sure they had.

That fall before moving to Connecticut, I was learning to be Nathan's mom. I was blessed with two awesome teachers: my mother and Carol. I adored them both, but occasionally became overwhelmed with the magnitude of my responsibilities. Those days we just tried to survive and deal with each trial as it came along.

One day Mom was trying to do some wall papering in the other room and Paul was bothering her, so she brought him into the living room, sat him down on the floor beside me, and shut the door. I was pretty depressed that day and couldn't stop the tears rolling down my cheeks, nor could I move. Neither of us said anything. Paul just crawled up into my lap and hugged me and we just sat there and rocked in the rocking chair for a long time. He was so sensitive to me and I was so happy to have someone to hold!!

I spent the fall with the two boys at my parent's house while Hank made the arrangements to move our family to Groton. When military housing became available it was January, a cold month to move, but we were both so anxious to be together that the weather didn't matter. I'm sure my parents were also looking forward to getting their lives back to normal.

Carol was a constant in our lives that fall and I don't know what I would have done without her. She definitely enriched our lives and I will forever be grateful to her for all her help and expertise in the care of my new baby. Carol's family continued living next door to my parents for about a year and then they moved. I felt privileged to have known her and to have her for a neighbor those first few months of Nathan's life. She definitely was our angel next door!

CHAPTER SIX

MOVING TO CONNECTICUT

My brother Sam and his wife Nancy, who lived in South Blue Hill had a pick-up truck. So when it came time to move to Groton, the plan was for them to drive me there. At the time Hank was packing up our belongings in Hawaii, he hadn't been assigned housing in Groton. When our things arrived at my parents' house we stored everything in one room. I was fortunate that Sam's pick-up would hold all of our possessions. We owned very little furniture but plenty of stuff.

Hank was sent to the barracks in New London in January, where he was now stationed. As soon as he called to say we had been assigned housing I made the arrangements to go, with my brother's help. Sam helped me pack all my household goods on the truck. His pick-up was loaded! We even had a new queen-sized mattress on top that was well covered to protect it from the weather.

My plan was for Paul to stay in Blue Hill with his grandparents. We had taken Nathan to Boston Children's Hospital earlier that week because of skin "break-down" around the stoma. It was so hard to keep that area clean enough for the skin to stay healthy. At that time, the doctors needed to give him a check-up so we would pick him up on the way back to Maine.

The call came and Hank was ready for us to come. He would meet us at 16 Spruce Lane, Groton, Connecticut, our new address. He took a few days off so we could get the house furnished before we brought the kids to their new home.

The truck was packed, we were ready, and I was filled with anticipation of our new life in our first house together as a family. Hank and I would spend most of the week buying furniture. To date, our furnishings consisted of baby items. We had a crib and a rocking chair, and my parents gave us a drop-leaf table to use for a changing table for Nathan. It was perfect because the top was wide enough for me to put all the supplies back where he couldn't reach, and still have room for a changing pad. I was able to attach a little mobile to the end of the table for Nathan to watch during the diaper changes. The little animals dangling over his head gave him some entertainment.

The weather report said "a possibility of snow". Everyone in New England knows what that means! But we were young and excited to go on this trip, so off we went. By the time we got to Bath the snow was really coming down. Sam got confused and went down the exit ramp just across the bridge. After a little slip and slide around the area, we found our way back on to Route 1.

Nancy grew up in West Newbury, Massachusetts, and knew a friend we could stay with for the night. So we went to this quaint little cottage surrounded with trees laden with snow. Mrs. Walker, who was probably all of eighty and lived alone, was so pleased to have us. We certainly were thankful to have a place to rest for the night! The little cottage had a cozy wood stove which made us particularly comfortable after travelling in stormy weather most of the day. I also remember the old-fashioned latch doors in that house. The whole place was so charming and welcoming, as was our hostess. After a bowl of hot chowder we were all so tired we went right to bed.

The morning sun woke us up early and after a hearty breakfast, cheerful conversation with Mrs. Walker, and many, many thanks, we were on our way. It had stopped snowing sometime in the night so we only had about six inches for the truck to negotiate a way out of the unplowed driveway. I felt so grateful for this extraordinarily beautiful day we were given to travel to Connecticut.

My heart was full and so happy to be on our way to my new home. This would be the place I dreamed of, and anticipated making a wonderful home for my little family. There would be ups and downs with Nathan's health issues but still I felt I'd been given such a gift: two beautiful, happy children. And I looked forward to the challenge of making this home especially warm and happy for them and my husband. Mostly I was looking forward to a normal family life with all of us together again; dreaming of a future with fewer trips to the hospital.

It turned out to be a beautiful second half of the journey. After a light snow the earth looked so fresh and clean while the sun danced on it as we drove down the highway. Sam and Nancy were fun to be with and we all had lots of stories and jokes to share on the trip south. The sun was melting the snow quickly and the roads were clearing as we traveled.

Back in Hawaii, Hank and I had bought a Chevy Nova. At the time, we didn't think much about the fact it didn't have a heater. We didn't consider that part of the world would never need a heater so most cars in Hawaii had none. Hank arranged for the car to be shipped to New London, where it now very much needed a heater, so Sam helped me get one from a junk yard in Maine and we brought it with us on the truck.

Early in the afternoon we arrived at Spruce Lane. Hank was there to meet us in that cold Chevy from Hawaii. It was particularly challenging for him to drive, not only because of tires made for Hawaiian roads, but now he had to drive with the window rolled down and his hand outside spraying a can of de-icer as he drove unfamiliar roads. At first the whole thing seemed comical, but soon we saw it was a serious problem that we had never anticipated. It was extremely cold travelling like that.

All afternoon the four of us worked hard unpacking the truck. Then Sam and Nancy left and we were alone to unpack the boxes and put things away the best we could with no furniture. I managed to put a few dishes in the cupboards and a few towels in the bathroom so we wouldn't have to start hunting when we first woke up. We found some blankets in a box and made a make-shift bed until we could actually buy one. Hank was much too tired that night to put the heater in the car so he decided to do it first thing in the morning. Great plan! There was no garage so he left the heater on the back steps.

When morning came we were incredibly disappointed to find the heater was gone! It never occurred to us that anyone would come up to our steps and take a car heater. We never knew who took it but here we were, ready to go furniture shopping in a car with no heat. To say the least, we both were becoming weary of this ordeal. To make matters worse, we didn't have any extra money to buy a heater. Hank knew people on base and asked someone where the local junk yard was. He walked through it until he found a new heater, which he installed completely by himself, but not before we spent a couple days shopping in a cold vehicle with the wind blowing in the windows!

Fortunately we had good luck shopping and quickly picked out washer, dryer, bed and two bureaus. We also found a dining room table with six chairs and a couch for the living room. Oh yes, we found a bedroom set for us that lasted twenty years of moving in the military service.

Finally the heater was put in the car, the house was ready, and all that was missing was the phone hook-up and two little boys. There were no cell phones in the seventies, so we hadn't been able to communicate with the boys or our family for a few days. Consequently, we were really missing them. It was time to get Nathan in Boston and head for Maine so we decided to call the hospital to see if Nathan was well enough to go home with us. This phone call was made on a pay phone in an inside corner of a Dunkin' Donuts very near our house. We had just bought a dozen donuts and for some reason I was holding them when I called the hospital. The doctor was available to talk to me and said Nathan was doing fine, so we could pick him up the next day at the designated time. My relief at hearing that good news was short lived. In the next breath, the doctor said "I just want you to be aware we have done tests and we're certain he has a problem with his heart. We don't know the extent of it yet but we will be watching him carefully." That was enough. It had been a trying week and this was basically the last straw for me. I just lost it right there with people all around me. The donuts went flying and I started sobbing and Hank took the phone and finished the conversation with the doctor. People were so kind to us and cleaned up the mess I had made. The clerk gave us another dozen for which I had totally lost my appetite.

A restless night's sleep and we were on our way to Boston. My dreams of happy, healthy children were once again on hold. The words of Dr. Bell, our first doctor in Portland, kept ringing in my ears: " There'll be a series of surgeries." It seemed like such a gloomy diagnosis; I couldn't fathom that concept. This would be one more example where we'd just have to take one episode at a time.

The ride was once again long and sober as we pondered the future. When we arrived at the hospital they had Nathan ready for us to take. He was so little and vulnerable and yet one look at him and my heart was on fire. I just picked him up and held him, thinking only of what a wonderful life he would have. Even at this early age he was an extraordinary little person and had all kinds of powers to win your heart. As I held him I just felt, all's right with the world, he's home with us! After getting Nathan, we traveled to Blue Hill where we spent a couple days before returning to finally start our life as a family together on Spruce Lane.

CHAPTER SEVEN

LONELINESS

Connecticut was a different experience for us. It was a cold, snowy winter and although we were in a neighborhood of houses spaced very close beside each other, I felt very isolated. Paul was now an active toddler and loved going outside no matter what the weather happened to be. When possible I would take him out to play in the snow. He loved making a snowman or just being in the snow. Nathan was just four months old and still required a lot of attention from me and the doctors. The majority of our outings that first winter were to the dispensary or commissary on base.

We began to feel comfortable in our new home on Spruce Lane. The home was a ranch style house with three bedrooms, a living room / dining area and small kitchen which contained our washer and dryer. A door between kitchen and dining room was occasionally closed while I made donuts, if I were so inspired. As good as they smelled cooking, they did fill the house with the odor of hot fat. With the kitchen door closed there would be no spreading of the grease smell through the house or worry about children and hot fat!

The house was in military housing and I felt very blessed to have a whole house to ourselves after living in a three room apartment. The arrangement of the house gave us much more room and each boy had his own bedroom, which was helpful to keep Paul out of Nathan's room, where he might be tempted to get into the creams and supplies there. Later in the spring we were able to use the large backyard which had a fence around it. We purchased a swing set for Paul and set up a sand box play area in the summer for him (and Nathan when he was old enough to play without eating the dirt!)

Once we were settled into our routine of Hank going to work early every day and the boys and I adjusting to the surroundings, I began to feel that old feeling of loneliness creeping back. It was hard to meet our neighbors, at this time of year there weren't many people outside. None of the people on Hank's ship had families in our housing area therefore I knew nobody in Connecticut.

Loneliness had come to call before. This wasn't my first time of dealing with that dreaded feeling. Hawaii was an absolutely gorgeous place to live and I will forever be grateful for that opportunity. The long sunny days and warm breezes kept a smile on your face most of the time. But when family and friends were far away and Hank was out to sea so much, gloomy times crept in. Hank left for Westpac seven weeks after Paul was born. I understood he would be gone for seven months and prepared myself for the long separation.

To ward off loneliness I met with some other Navy wives. We got together for occasional meals and times at the beach where they would help watch Paul while I went for a swim. Just to see people and get out of our little apartment would enrich and boost our spirits. Paul loved to go for a ride in the stroller, therefore I'd plan an outing for us almost every day. Sometimes it was a simple walk around the block or down to the park where we saw large goldfish swimming in a man-made pool. Beautiful flowers dotted the landscape wherever we went in Hawaii.

The loneliness that I was feeling here in Connecticut was very similar to that feeling of isolation I had in Hawaii. And yet this nagging ache inside felt more like the kind of loneliness a person wouldn't necessarily feel in his every-day life. Now I had a four-month old baby that could only be taken care of by Hank or me. The diaper change itself was too complicated to try to teach anybody that wouldn't be seeing him on a regular basis. My loneliness was not just the feeling of isolation but basic insecurity about my abilities. This child depended on me to take care of all his needs and keep him out of the hospital. "Looking back, I see I put that part on myself." Every time Nathan had to go back to the hospital for anything other than a scheduled surgery, I felt I'd failed. Encouraging each other at these times became Hanks' and my routine, because we both knew we'd done all we could.

Mothers with small children naturally get together and talk over problems they have with their kids' eating, behaviors, potty training, and so forth. All parents have those things in common. There just didn't seem to be anyone in my world that was dealing with the things before me. There was nobody there for me to call and ask, "What do you do about leakage through clothing by the ureterostomies?" or " How would you deal with a colostomy bag that came loose?" At the dispensaries, where we spent a lot of time, the doctors had not seen a child "built" just like mine. They did their best, and I always appreciated their suggestions, but several times they just didn't know, so had to send us to Boston Children's Hospital. I was so thankful we were only a couple of hours away from them.

One time I felt very insecure and called for a visiting nurse to see if she had some ideas that would help our situation. She came and talked to me for a while and saw how things were being done, and just said she thought I was doing fine. That was not what I needed at the time, but how could I expect someone who'd never dealt with a child with these particular problems to give me answers?

There is a kind of loneliness that is different from the kind that is common to all. I'd never known this kind of extreme loneliness. I felt inadequate at taking care of my baby, and missed having an adult to talk to. Hank seemed to be gone to work all the time. Now I felt like I was alone on an island. The days were long and lonely. My child needed me to know what to do for his very existence. Knowing all the answers to his needs was not in my experience. It was not just taking care of a new baby, but a baby that needed special attention to his body in ways most babies didn't.

I was not the only one feeling insecure caring for this baby with different needs. The doctors at the dispensary on base seemed quite challenged by his care. Whenever we went in with Nathan, appointment or not, waiting room full or not, they would take us right in immediately. They really were wonderful to us, and I definitely appreciated the support we received.

Hank remembers those stressful days when he would have to take Nathan to the dispensary on base after hours, when the doctor had to be specially called in. Hank apologized for making him come in just for us. The doctor told him, "Don't ever apologize for calling me in. I'll come anytime for your son." Because Nathan was so little when we lived in Groton, we were constantly taking him to the doctors, either on base or at Children's Hospital in Boston. The break-down of skin around Nathan's colostomy was the most common reason for visits to the hospital. The colostomy was high on his abdomen and the discharge would run down his skin until it made ridges where the skin broke away. Sometimes, it would take a weeks' hospitalization for that to heal. There was always pressure on Hank if he had to leave work for these occasions.

For example one time I brought Nathan in and the doctor wanted to keep him in the dispensary overnight while he treated him with a barium enema. He felt there was some blockage in Nathan's colon and this would help. It appeared to be the right thing at the time so we allowed it. The next day things weren't going as he expected so the doctor called me to come right in. He said he had called for a base ambulance for Nathan and wanted me to go with them to Boston Children's Hospital. Naturally, the idea was very upsetting to me but when I saw the panic in his face it alarmed me.

The two-hour ride was very nerve-racking. The ambulance driver was not sure of the area around the hospital in Boston and expected me to direct him. I was always the passenger, not the driver, whenever we took Nathan, so this added to my stress. My mind was sick with worry about Nathan, and the driver turning the siren on when we arrived in the city didn't help. By then it was dark, but the driver did manage to navigate his way to the hospital without my input, thankfully! When we drove into the emergency bay there was a doctor to attend to Nathan immediately. He reassured me everything would be okay, and that after the initial examination, they were taking him to a treatment room, and then to the pediatric ward. At that point it was time for me to step back and let the doctors take care of him; I would be able to go to him when he arrived on the ward. So I trusted and prayed. Nathan did well, and we were able to take him home in a couple days when Hank and Paul came to pick us up.

January was not a good month to meet new neighbors. It was so cold and windy that we only went out when we needed to. Then one day this lovely lady knocked on my door. I was so excited and eagerly invited her in to visit. She represented the local "Welcome Wagon" organization. Never having heard of it, I thought that sounded like the nicest kind of a name for an organization! I invited her in to sit. "Can I take your coat? Would you like coffee or tea?" She looked at me funny, as if she wanted to run out the door! Maybe she'd never met anyone quite as desperate for company. She said, "I just came to bring you this yardstick and some information about the area and welcome you to Groton." My reply was "Thank you so much. Where do you live?" She answered, "Not here; on the other side of town." With that she quickly exited, talking of the many other stops she had to make that day. I was terribly disappointed and didn't feel a bit welcomed to this town!

I longed for a friend who could understand and affirm my efforts once in a while. When Nathan was this little and needed me so much, I couldn't get out to church or any other social events. Nevertheless, there had to be a way to meet someone in this community, so I set my sights on my next door neighbor. This time I would have a strategy. Our kitchen doors, which had windows in them, faced each other. The two driveways were right beside each other. When Hank had gone to work, it was a clear view into her yard. Hence I watched for her to come out to get in her car, or throw her garbage in the cans out back. If I saw her, I'd open the door and give a wave and a friendly "Hi!" She tried to ignore me but I was determined. Eventually she responded and we got together for coffee. Bev and I became good friends and our children were close in ages. John and Paul became play buddies right away but Kelly and Nathan were too little to care about each other.

Ultimately Hank could see I needed some time away from the house, so he suggested I take a course to renew my teaching license. He would stay with the kids one night a week while I took a course in early childhood education. There were activities to do with preschool children, so Bev and I would get together with our kids. Once we made peanut butter and the kids helped with shelling peanuts. On a different occasion, we did a Teddy Bears' Picnic with them. Mainly the older boys enjoyed it. For me, it was so nice to have a supportive friend next door we could do things with. Bev was a wonderful friend and neighbor to us. We found we had things in common and enjoyed getting together for coffee or just a visit from time to time. At last I knew someone in our neighborhood. Besides being a friend, she went above and beyond friendship several times, when she took Paul for us while we needed to get Nathan to a hospital or dispensary. Many times I wondered what I ever would have done without the help and support of Bev.

At this time we were taking Nathan to Boston Children's Hospital, two hours away from us, for most of his major doctoring. It was a tough trip when we were taking a sick child for medical help and had a toddler fussing to go home. The times Bev helped us out by taking Paul was such a blessing. One time we were taking Nathan to a scheduled surgery in Boston and intended to take Paul along. The boys, already dressed, were waiting for Hank to get home from work. As I was in the bathroom down the hall, Paul went looking for me and came running down the hall and slipped on the hard-wood floor hitting his head hard on the door casing. Blood everywhere! As you can imagine he was crying a lot, which then upset Nathan so he came to see what was going on and crawled right through the blood. What a mess we all were! Hank arrived to find us in this tither. He took Paul immediately to the dispensary for stitches, while I cleaned Nathan up for the trip. This was one of the times Bev graciously agreed to have Paul while we were gone, with only a few minutes notice. That day Hank had happened to pick up a large stuffed alligator at the exchange. It was comforting to Paul so he clung to the toy while we were gone. This was one of many occurrences we were pulled in troublesome times, with two children needing you for two different reasons and not being able to be with both. This time it turned out well because we had a friend like Bev. Bev and I kept in touch over the years with Christmas Cards or a note.

Charleston, South Carolina, was our next station after Groton, Connecticut. Bev's husband also had received orders for the same place a few months later. Unfortunately, we had orders to leave Charleston even before Bev and her family had moved into housing.

Most of the times Nathan had to be admitted to the hospital was because of the breakdown of the skin around the stoma. While he was healing the medical staff would do tests related to his condition. VACTERL association affects individuals differently. For example, with Nathan's heart, the doctors would find new things, like a shadow they didn't understand, to watch out for at various examinations. At one time I was actually told that Nathan wouldn't walk. My mind immediately rejected that thought. We became a little concerned when he didn't walk around twelve months, like most children,

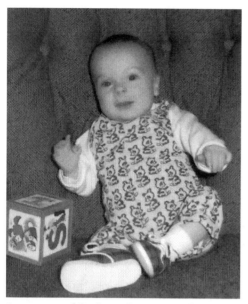

wondering if that doctor might be right. Thankfully, he started his toddling days at the age of eighteen months.

In spite of all Nathan went through as a baby and later in life, he was an extremely good – natured individual. After surgeries as an infant, I expected some fussiness, or chronic crying to indicate discomfort. It never happened with him. I was told by doctors that infants heal very fast and did experience that up close, later on in his care, when his body actually healed where it shouldn't have.

Nathan was generally a smiley, happy baby, as any other baby would have been. To see him you'd never guess he'd been through all that had happened to him. Nathan was never a demanding child. He certainly had plenty of reason to be, and no one would have faulted him for it. As he grew, we realized his personality more than made up for the physical deficiencies he was born with. His even – tempered, happy disposition won the hearts of the medical staff everywhere we went, as well as all the hearts of our family and friends.

*   *   *

Recently I was asked how I actually overcame the depression and loneliness that tried to control me during Nathan's early days. After thinking back over my life, I credit the way my parents raised us, as having a lot to do with how we handled tough times. My Mom would wake me up on a Saturday morning, throwing the window curtains open while singing "O What a Beautiful Morning!" from the musical Oklahoma. "Rise and shine!" she'd say, promising when my chores were done, I could go bicycling with my friend. She was always fair and usually a happy and upbeat person. She definitely was my example of how to live.

Also, from the earliest times of my childhood, we all went to church. We learned about the power of prayer, and loving God and others. As an adult whenever we moved in the military, I would visit the various churches in a community, until I found the Bible believing church that was right for my family. The most important thing in my life was, and is my relationship with God and my family. Because of what I learned in my childhood, I knew it would be up to me to find creative ways to live through the challenges of caring for someone with such health issues as Nathan had. In life everyone needs a sense of humor so always nurture that. It got us through many very serious times.

CHAPTER EIGHT

THE POWER OF LOVE

Hank was a First Class Sonar Technician stationed on a tender, the *USS Fulton* in New London, CT. In order to go to work he had to cross the river between Groton and New London. Many times he would leave the car with me and walk to work if I needed to drive Nathan to the dispensary, we only had the one vehicle. The shortest way was to walk on the train bridge on its narrow walkway. If a train came by, he stood as close to the hand rail as possible. No fencing existed between him and the train, which made windy days particularly uncomfortable.

Over the years I have often thought back on those days when he selflessly walked to work, crossing the river on a train bridge. He did that the two years we lived in Groton, and some of those days were in the bitter cold of New England winter. He never gave it a second thought and never complained or talked about it.

One morning Nathan woke up breathing strangely and coughing. It sounded like a cold but the breathing was worrisome. So that morning Hank walked and left the car for me to take Nathan in to see the doctor.

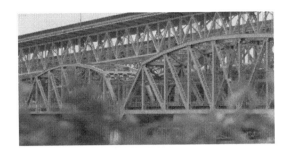

Train bridge: New London & Groton, CT

I bundled both boys for the cold weather and we headed out for the dispensary. After examining him the doctor insisted we take Nathan to the hospital immediately. He suggested we consider Boston Children's or Yale New Haven. Hank and I chose Yale New Haven because Nathan's cardiologist, Dr. Whittermore, was affiliated with that hospital. We had been taking Nathan to her at the heart clinic in Norwich, and she had seen a shadow on his heart X-ray which she didn't understand. Dr. Whittermore informed us that at some point she wanted to do a catheterization on Nathan's heart. Hank and I really didn't understand what that meant other than it was a test. Dr. Whittermore, an older woman, and very experienced, assured us she would be there at Yale New Haven, and personally look out for Nathan. When he was feeling better she would do the catheterization. In time we learned that it was a rather complex test. They needed to go with a tube up through a vein in his groin to his heart. Had we known how invasive it was, I doubt we would have allowed it on such a tiny body.

Paul was now two, and his favorite toy was a Humpty Dumpty shaped like a child's pillow with arms and legs that had no stuffing. His constant companion, Paul carried it everywhere. He also loved two old sailor hats his Dad had given him and usually wore them together.

That afternoon when Hank got home, I had the boys all ready for the trip to New Haven. Paul had his two hats on and Humpty Dumpty in tow. It was a long ride and Nathan's breathing seemed more labored than before, which caused great worry.

When we arrived, he was immediately taken to be checked. They put him in an oxygen tent right away to help his breathing. The initial diagnosis was that he probably had bronchitis. I explained to the nurses that the skin around his stoma was breaking down and would need special attention. They also received an explanation of how I had been taught to care for the skin that needed attention around his stoma, as well as the ureterostomies. The creams they would need were left with the nurses.

When the staff was working on Nathan, they asked us to sit in the waiting room. Hank couldn't sit, so he paced. A student came up to me and introduced himself and asked if he could interview me about Nathan's condition. I said, "Of course!" I was happy to give more information so they'd know how to treat him. I sat with the young man for an hour and told all of Nathan's story since he had been born four months ago. The student was taking notes the whole time and seemed to find Nathan's case to be very interesting. Shockingly, ten days later I met this young man in the hall and he just looked away without even speaking to me. I was horrified! With what kind of people had we left our baby?

Before we left the hospital, Dr. Whittermore briefly spoke to us, and assured us Nathan would be fine. She promised to personally check on him. We were given phone numbers to call to see how he was doing. By then it was very late and we were trying to keep a two year old happy while worrying about whether Nathan was receiving the care he needed.

We kept in touch with the hospital all week and then received a call from Dr. Whittermore that he was out of the oxygen tent and eating, so she would do the catheterization. Later she called to tell us the test didn't reveal much but she would like to continue to monitor his progress. I felt confident that Nathan was being well taken care of because she was there checking on him. We agreed to pick him up the following Saturday.

Once the day came, we arrived on the pediatric ward to find no one around. A nurse came out and said she'd get the doctor on duty. He was very young and said he was filling in for another doctor. This wasn't his ward. He told us we could visit with Nathan. This doctor didn't know we were there to take Nathan home.

Paul wasn't allowed on the ward with the sick children so Hank stayed with him while I went in. It was a ward of cribs, all having the same gray, institutional look about them. Some of them were empty. I looked in all the cribs that had babies in them and didn't see Nathan. I walked around the whole room and couldn't find him. As I started back towards the door, at eye level on the end of a crib there was a tag that said Nathan Fenders. My heart started pounding and tears welled up in my eyes as I looked at the child that didn't look like mine. He did not recognize me when I spoke. His little eyes darted from side to side and back at me as if to say, "What are you going to do to me now!" He was lying on his side naked with his hands wrapped in a diaper that was pinned to the sheet, and his feet were secured in the same fashion. The bile from his stoma was oozing down the side of his abdomen causing the skin to erode. He had needle marks on his ankles, and arms, and even on his forehead. I began to wonder if they had even given him a bottle at all; he looked so thin and frail. I felt myself becoming sick. How could we have trusted these people? What was this place?

I went out to stay with Paul so Hank could go see him, and he didn't recognize him either. I berated the poor doctor who was subbing for a friend, until I realized he had no control of this situation.

Hank came out as upset as I was so all I could see to do, I did: I went back to that child, my Nathan, and gently and carefully released him from his bondage, cleaned him thoroughly, and diapered and dressed him. There was one nurse there with a toddler who had been running around the ward. She put all her attention on this seemingly healthy child while I was seething inside. She asked me, "Can I help you?" My reply was, "I think you've done enough!" After detailed instruction to the nurses on how to care for the openings on Nathan's abdomen, it was obvious to me they had ignored my words. In the stand drawer by Nathan's crib I found the tube of cream I'd left for them to use on his ureterostomies. The cover was off and it looked like it had been just thrown in. Weren't they the professionals? Didn't they know about cleanliness? All this just added to my mixed emotions of anger and heartbreak!

Whenever I remember that day, I actually begin to tremble inside and feel sick to my stomach. How could we have left him there for ten days for them to prick, poke, and ignore until he was afraid of everyone who came near? At the time, there was no option and we were so young and ignorant about medical matters that we had to trust the doctors. We were still learning how to care for this incredibly sick child.

After dressing him, I held him tight as we left the hospital. The doctor on duty tried to stop us: "You can't just take him without his doctor discharging him!" My reply to him was, "Watch me!" We walked out of that hospital and didn't look back.

I had brought a bottle with me to feed Nathan on the way home. He drank a little and fell asleep. Thank God it was Saturday and Hank was home for the weekend. We held that child constantly, and we talked to him and we loved him. His little eyes continued to dart around as if he didn't trust us. We couldn't get him to smile nor would he cry.

That whole weekend, whenever he wasn't being fed or sleeping, I was rocking him and singing to him. The fear that we wouldn't be able to get him back to normal was overtaking my thoughts. The first night while rocking him, holding, and singing to him whenever he was awake, there still was no response from my frightened little child. Finally, when he fell asleep for the night, exhaustion took over my body and I went to bed and sobbed. I told Hank, "I think we're going to lose him this time. He doesn't respond to anything." Hank held me tight and said, "We're not going to lose him. Nathan will come around. He's going to be OK." So I held that thought in my head and my heart and fell asleep knowing that God had given me the right man for a husband. Hank was always there to help when things became really rough. These were some of the toughest days we had to go through, but it kept us close and, over the years, even closer. Still, it was a lonely time for each of us when all we had was each other.

We continued our routine with Nathan: holding, talking, singing, and rocking him every waking moment. Finally, after two long days he smiled! Our whole family was so excited, our baby was back. We just kept loving him until he had to smile at us! That was our sign he would be alright.

CHAPTER NINE

MY YOUTH

It has been said that your experiences in life build on one another in preparation for what lies ahead. I've thought about this in terms of my life as the mother of a child with VACTERL association. There were three major parts of my youth that I believe contributed to my ability to care for a child like my Nathan. They were my bouts with ear infections, the Girl Scout years, and my piano lessons which lead to my teaching career.

My mother told me that as an infant, I had had severe ear infections. She said she actually worried that I could die or the infections would leave me deaf. When my ears became infected, the fever caused my body to become lethargic and it frightened her. These infections, all of which took place before antibiotics were widely used, continued throughout my early years. At about age twelve, doctors were able to give me penicillin in a needle.

Sometimes when I was out of school for many days at a time with the ear infections, my mother would take time off from work to stay home with me. I could feel the pressure build up in my ear and then there'd be a pop and pus would drain from my ear. Mom gave me one of my fathers' pocket handkerchiefs to catch it. Waking up from a sleep, I'd hear a whistling tea kettle and scream for Mom to take it off the stove. That's when she told me she'd thrown that tea kettle away weeks ago. It was horrible when the whistle in my ear wouldn't stop.

Mom tried to spend time with me because she realized I was alone in my room for days on end. From my second story bedroom window my mother would hang out the laundry, on a pulley line my father had put from the corner of the window to the top of the barn roof. My mother would sit on the window sill and lean out the window to hang out clothes. Sometimes she would take them in and leave them in a chair by the window. I woke up in the night to see what looked like someone sitting in that chair. I was so scared I'd pull the covers over my head. After I'd worked myself into a frenzy I would scream for my parents. Their room was next to mine and Mom came running thinking it was my ears again. When I told her the problem she said to me, "Anytime you feel afraid you look at what makes you afraid. Next time you turn your light on and see it is just a pile of clothes." Now, when my grandkids tell me they are afraid of something, I tell them to go look: "Check under your bed if you think there's a boogie man there." Mom taught me a very important lesson, which is: "Face your fears", and I hope to pass that on to my children and grandkids.

In the seventh grade my desk was placed in front of the teacher so I could hear her. The infections kept me out of school many days that year. One day I noticed several students behind me were pointing at the teacher. When I looked at her, she was talking to me but I couldn't hear her words. They sent me home that day and my parents took me to an ear specialist soon after that. The doctor said he would need to do surgery on the mastoid bone of my left ear. However, by the time I went for the surgery I was pretty deaf in both ears. I remember when they admitted me, the doctor kept trying to tell me he wanted to take some blood from my arm. I couldn't hear a word he said. Somehow, my mother knew how to talk to me and she'd get right in my face and explain what he had said. It made all the difference and I depended on her completely.

My parents were always supportive of me but the hospital was an hour's drive away from home. Three brothers at home also needed them. It was February and the snow storms were still happening frequently. There were days they just couldn't come to see me and those were very long lonely days. The nurses were nice to me but busy with many children. I had been put on a children's ward although I was no longer a child. The alternative would be a bed in the hallway. There was a small room with two beds just off the children's ward that they let me have. The walls were painted with cowboys on bucking broncos; this was before there was a TV in every hospital room. It seemed twice a day my meal tray would have mashed potatoes and I wanted so badly for that cowboy in front of me to meet those potatoes! I did receive a lot of cards from home and looked forward every day to those caring messages. My Aunt Eleanor sent up a "sunshine basket" filled with happy little goodies to cheer me up. It was the first time I'd ever heard of a sunshine basket, and it certainly did make me feel loved. She was very close to our family, and always a favorite aunt for my brothers and me.

After surgery on the left ear, I remained nine days in the hospital and received thirty six shots of penicillin . Surprisingly I was able to hear in both ears immediately after waking from the surgery. That seemed strange because I was deaf in both ears, but only one was operated on and yet I could hear in both. I always felt that was God's hand on me.

Nathan was about eleven when he had his open heart surgery, close to the age I was when I had my ear operated on. He had a hole in the top of his heart that needed to be patched, plus an extra artery that needed to be clamped off. The surgery was very successful, and when he was put back into a room, the nurses kept asking if he needed pain medication. He always refused. I told him it was fine to take them but he insisted he didn't have pain. As with my ear surgery, again, I felt God's hand on him.

Later in my seventh grade year, something very exciting happened to change my life. My mother found a new piano teacher for me, since my last one had moved away. John Dethier was a retired school music teacher, organist, and originally, a concert pianist from Belgium. He would only accept students who had taken lessons for at least two years, and I met the requirements. I was so excited to be back taking lessons, and he was just amazing as a teacher! My pursuit of the piano continued with Mr. Dethier right through my college years. He taught me so many things that my lessons never seemed to be limited to one hour. Many Saturday mornings I walked a mile up Green's Hill in Blue Hill for a nine o'clock lesson, and returned home in time for lunch. After we'd been over all my music for the lesson, we sometimes would go to his dining room table and he'd teach me theory. He really gave me a head start for theory class in college. As I left my teacher's house to walk down the hill I looked off in the distance, over roof tops to open fields and saw the ocean with little islands in the bay. On the horizon I could see the "Sleeping Giant" of Bar Harbor. My heart was overflowing with love for this small town called Blue Hill, and the music I anticipated working on. At that moment I was sure that I was the luckiest girl in the world; it took gravity to keep me from skipping downhill. That very afternoon I would sit at the piano and go over all my music to be sure I remembered everything Mr. Dethier said. I had so much passion for playing that I spent all my free time practicing. It was my happiness, as trying to reach the goals Mr. Dethier set for me each week challenged me, almost to the point of obsession.

The stamina I learned from those hours of practice, which eventually grew to six or seven hours a day in college, contributed to my determination in life. It became important to do my absolute best, and when recital time came in college my oboe friend, Sandy, and I were the second two in the history of the college to do our graduation recitals our junior year. The requirement was one hour of memorized music, which terrified both of us because we did not memorize easily. Sandy and I had seen too many students fail to graduate because they were unable to fulfill the recital obligation, so to be safe we decided to start a year early. It took a solid year to prepare for that, and Sandy and I performed the same day, me in the afternoon and her in the evening. We both passed the requirement with flying colors! I went on to do three more public recitals; the last one was in 1981 when I had three little boys. The piano taught me focus and control of my mind and hands (and, later my feet for the organ). Playing the piano was always a privilege and pleasure in my life.

The third part of my life that gave me preparation for being Nathan's Mom was Scouting. I was a Girl Scout from a very young age right through high school. My junior year of high school , after writing an essay of application, I was chosen for a one - month trip to Washington State. It was a special honor for a small- town girl who had never been out of the state of Maine or flown on an airplane. My responsibility was to make all the arrangements myself so I obtained the addresses of the other two girls from New England going on this trip. After writing to them the plan was that I would take the train to Seattle with another scout from Connecticut. Coming home, I would fly with a girl from Concord, Massachusetts .

My parents drove me to Springfield, Connecticut to meet my travelling friend, Vera. Her parents were very kind and invited my parents to spend the night. The next day Vera and I set out for four days of travelling to Seattle on the train. Once we were settled on the train, we decided to take a walk around to see what it was like. Upon arriving at the dining car, we decided to sit and have a Coke. In the late sixties they were about twenty-five cents a can. When the waiter brought it and asked each of us for $2.50 I laughed out loud! He didn't! From then on we kept a close watch on the prices so our money would last the whole trip. During this train adventure trip, we had our own little room with comfortable seats that made into beds at night. The train also had a Scenic Car, in which passengers could go to an upper level to watch the beautiful landscape of the many states we passed through. From Connecticut to Seattle we saw many panoramic views that we would never have seen if we flew both ways.

A local Girl Scout Leader was there to meet us at the train station in Seattle. She took us to do a little sight- seeing around the Space Needle, where the World's Fair had been a couple years before. After the tour, she delivered us to the campsite in Carnation, Washington. Girl Scouts from all over the country greeted us. Carnation would be our headquarters the whole time we were there.

Each Scout was assigned specific jobs. We would leave with different local scout leaders to do our various jobs. My job was to train scout leaders for camping. Neither of my traveling buddies had the same assignment, so I was put with another girl. I'd done a lot of camping with my family, as well as with other Scouts but the biggest challenge for us in this environment was the rain. It rained every day the whole month of August. Even the days the sun came out we hardly had time to get the cameras before it was raining again! My co-worker Scout didn't have much experience camping. The leaders we took with their troop had little or no camping skills, and the girls were eager but not necessarily ready for the work that was required of them. The success of the camping week seemed to be left up to me so this event became one of the first leadership projects in my life. When things didn't go well, like the constant rain, and the whining of wet ten-year- old Scouts and a complaining co-worker, we just kept working at it. We were even able to build fires with soaking wet cedar. Problem solving became a big part of our daily routine, where we learned to make do with whatever we had to work with. We also had to be patient and kind in every miserable situation we found ourselves.

I believe these three major parts of my life as a young person shaped and prepared me to be the kind of parent Nathan needed. As a child with ear infections, I learned to trust doctors, my parents, and God for my health. On the Scout trip there were lessons of organization, patience with others, and tolerance for tough situations, and perseverance when others became discouraged. The piano taught discipline, which was not automatic. I could discipline myself to practice but when the piece was very difficult, it was harder to stay with it. No matter how hard the piece was, there was never an option to skip it. One of my recital pieces in college was so difficult that I begged the teacher to give me something different, which of course, he wouldn't. By the time of the recital it had become my favorite thing to play.

Most especially the person I chose to marry made a huge difference in the outcomes of our lives. Nathan's Dad had many attributes that made him the perfect candidate to be the Dad of a child with many needs. Hank was military and that's how his mind worked. If we were scheduled to be at Boston Children's Hospital for Nathan's surgery on a Tuesday at 12 o'clock they had better be ready for us! There was an incident just like that when the nurses weren't ready for Nathan. Hank, remembering that our first surgeon, Dr. Bell, had told us to always talk to the person in charge, made that demand. It was noontime and we were lucky to get to speak to the nurse in charge. He let them know we were taking our two boys out for lunch and when we came back, that room had better be ready. Believe me, it was! When we saw the doctor later that afternoon, he laughed and said "I hear you got things going around here."

Hank had the ability and desire to figure things out. He had studied engineering and math and had a logical mind, always trying to "trouble shoot" any problems that arose. He taught every one of our kids math so they had no problems with it in school. He's the kind of person who will take time to read directions when putting things together. Hank found some plans for making a wall unit in our first house in Connecticut. It took up one whole wall and held our stereo equipment, TV, records, books and anything else we needed to put there. He painted the frame gold and the shelves blue. It could be taken apart, and we used it for every move until we retired in our own home. There he put it in the basement to be for storage. There were so many times he would see a need and figure out a solution.

Nathan's dad always put his family first. When we were going through the rough times and needed to get Nathan to a hospital Hank would work something out at his ship so he could get off early. He helped me with every part of Nathan's care that he possibly could. We definitely worked as a team during those difficult times in Nathan's life.

CHAPTER TEN

THE BAG

In the spring of his first year we took Nathan to Boston Children's Hospital for a check-up with our surgeon, Dr. Eraklis. Hank and I were very anxious to hear when the colostomy, and the ureterostomies would be closed. Nathan was growing all the time, and the diaper changes were long and hard to do. As he grew and ate more, these half hour changes became more frequent. There were no Pampers that would fit and stop leaks onto outer garments. I tried plastic pants to cover the ureterostomies but he was rolling more and they hardly reached far enough to do any good. It was a constant battle. The surgery couldn't happen soon enough for me, but Nathan was only six months old and the doctor said he wouldn't consider surgery before he was a year old.

However, Dr. Eraklis did have a bit of encouraging news. A company was making colostomy bags a little smaller for children. The doctor said it was totally up to us if we wanted to use the bags, but if we did, we would have to commit to them for a period of time. If they did not work out well, we could go back to what we were doing. Dr. Eraklis did not try to influence our decision because it was so new. Hank and I talked about it and decided it sounded like a good idea. There was a ring that would fit around the stoma and attach to his skin. The good part was that none of the fecal material would touch his skin, so there would be better protection . We liked the sound of that, and so we decided to try it out. The doctor showed us how to put the bag on, which had to be done in such a particular way that it took two people. Twice a day Hank and I put this bag over Nathan's stoma, once in the morning and once at night. The ureterostomies still had to be taken care of with cream and gauze pads and the cloth diaper wrapped around his abdomen.

It wasn't an easy procedure, but together we were able to do this every day. The comical part was when Nathan broke wind, it filled his bag with air. So sometimes I had a "fat" little boy that was full of air! I tried to put larger - sized outfits on him but at times he looked like a real life Humpty Dumpty!

We continued to work with the bags the best we could for the next few months before his pull-thru surgery. We bought the smallest size bags and tried to make them work, but even they were really too large for him. We had many frustrating times with the bag, and sometimes it took us longer than expected to put it on.

One day the unexpected happened. The bag came off while Hank was at work and I was alone with the boys. My neighbor, Bev, was gone, so I panicked. Then I remembered Bev had once introduced me to her neighbor. We had met briefly, and she was the only person I knew to ask for help. Jane lived a stone's throw from Bev's house; I could easily see her house directly across the cul de sac from me. Since there seemed to be no alternative, I decided to humble myself and ask for help.

Paul was sound asleep taking a nap; Nathan was safely in his crib and I ran for help. My poor neighbor was cooking bacon for her husband's lunch. Apologizing for interrupting them, I begged! Jane reluctantly came and helped me. I don't know if she'd ever seen a colostomy but she didn't say a word. She did exactly what she was told to do and we got the bag back on to Nathan all secure. She left; I never saw her again and I'm willing to bet she didn't eat lunch that day! I often wondered what Jane was thinking as we did this. After explaining the situation to her she still wasn't saying anything.

When you think of the word "neighborly" or "being neighborly", I guess you wouldn't expect to be asked to help with a colostomy bag on a baby. God bless those who would willingly help a stranger do a task that they couldn't ever have imagined.

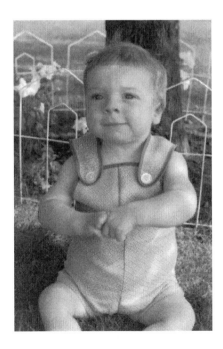

CHAPTER ELEVEN

SUMMER IN BLUE HILL

Summertime in 1974 we decided to go to Maine for a vacation, so Hank drove us to my parents' house. He left us for a week and then came back and took leave for the second week, so he could actually have a little vacation time as well.

This was the first summer we started our tradition of going to visit grandparents in Blue Hill. My mother still did bookkeeping at her office in her house. She had two doors to shut herself in so little people wouldn't interrupt her work. At this time, Paul was two and a half and running everywhere. Nathan was still wearing the colostomy bag and that really slowed his development as far as crawling on his hands and knees. The bag seemed to be too much padding on his abdomen. At least I knew where he was all the time: right where I put him! I would sit him in a comfortable place with lots of toys for him to play with. Of course, for entertainment, he had Paul running and tumbling all around him. Nathan was completely happy watching his brother. The more he laughed, the more Paul would put on a show for him.

Being home in Blue Hill felt like relief to me. Mom and Dad both had to work but, Mom worked from home, she could take a coffee break anytime she wanted to. My mom was such great company and comfort for me; we were always close and whenever we got together, we could talk for hours.

Dad, was my rock, a man of very few words, but when he spoke there was something to listen to. He always gave me encouragement and supported whatever I was doing, whether it was school related, a recital or the present challenge of caring for Nathan's needs. When I became discouraged and down at the mouth, and couldn't seem to see the forest for the trees, Dad would say something encouraging. Many times he said, "Nathan will be healthy again" or "He's going to be okay." He always said it in a tone of voice that sounded like he knew something nobody else did. I personally believe it was his direct line to the Heavenly Father-because Dad was definitely right.

During Hank's vacation week with us, we took the boys to the beach in East Blue Hill. Curtis Cove has a picturesque beach I'd spent many summer days on as a child. Many Sundays after church we'd put our bathing suits on and Mom would make a picnic and we'd spend the whole afternoon at the beach with cousins. A special memory was that the picnic always seemed to be plenty ample for lunch and supper, if we decided to stay . Everything depended on the weather, the tide, and how much the four of us kids would tease to stay! Usually Dad would build a fire right on the rocks and cut some narrow branches from a nearby tree. We'd stick a hot dog on these green branches to cook over the fire. Occasionally Mom brought marshmallows as well. These afternoons were the only times my parents would allow us to have root beer and orange soda, until we were older. In our pre-teens, it was a special treat to have popcorn and soda on Saturday nights while watching a TV show.

Now I was bringing my own children to this exceptional place of many happy memories. They were too young to enjoy the soda yet, but the excitement of being at the ocean would definitely call them back many times.

The tide on this particular beach would come up to large rocks close to the tree line where we could sit in either shade or sun. When it went out, it would go off the rocks completely, down the sand the length of a football field at the lowest tide. The day Hank and I took the boys, there was a lot of sand on the beach so we could go out a long distance and still be in shallow water. It was smoldering hot and we all wanted to get in the water! Hank had made a little wooden sailboat for Paul. He tied a string on it and sailed it out quite a ways before pulling it back. Paul just loved it and went in the shallow water chasing it as Hank pulled it around for him. I would hold Nathan and dip his feet in the water so he could see what the excitement was all about.

That vacation week we were able to visit with my brother, Jon and his wife, Sandy. They had Peter, a little younger than Paul, and Tobey was a baby. Sandy and Jon were married while we were in Hawaii so I was just getting to know my sister-in-law. We had so much in common, and it was really nice to have another young mom to talk to.

Hank had something special he wanted to do this vacation. One day he asked my mother if she'd watch the kids for a while so we could go out to lunch. Lunch! What an intriguing idea! Go out - just the two of us? It seemed such a long time since we'd done anything without kids. I couldn't even imagine! We weren't gone very long and all I could think of was getting back to the kids. Since leaving Blue Hill, our conversation had been completely about them.

After lunch Hank wanted to take me to a place he had in mind, which to my surprise was a music store. Inside the building was a whole first floor of pianos. They were so beautiful that I wanted to try them all! A sea of baby grands, Steinways, Wurlitzers and, a new name in pianos, Yamaha, filled my senses as they beckoned for someone to play them. Suddenly I thought, "Is this a cruel joke?" None of them were in our budget! But, I'd never known my husband to do anything that mean. When he said for me to try some of them, I knew he was serious. A light brown Wurlitzer Console summoned me, and I fell in love with the touch and sound of it. When Hank told the salesperson, "We'll take it," I couldn't believe my ears! It was something I'd missed for so long but didn't dare think about ever getting - certainly not in the near future.

The Chickering Square Grand that I grew up practicing on had been given away. Thankfully, it was given by my parents to a young girl who wouldn't have been able to afford a piano, and who also went on to become quite an accomplished pianist. So the sting of losing my childhood friend was eased. And now the joy of choosing my new instrument filled my heart.

Hank had just received a bonus that he hadn't told me about and he'd decided to put it all into this piano for me. It was totally overwhelming to think he would do this just for me and I would have my own piano again! A piano was not even on my radar. I couldn't begin to think of anything like that. We had so many other things to focus on for the family. And yet, my husband must have recognized those long, lonely days in Connecticut when I was so desperately trying to find a friend. So we rented a U-Haul and took it back to Spruce Lane with us. It certainly gave me a reason to look forward to going back to Groton. I could hardly wait to start playing again!

In future summers, we continued to come to Maine, many times for the whole summer. The boys looked forward to being in Blue Hill and receiving lots of attention from their grandparents. Summertime brought many new adventures into the lives of my children. Aunts and uncles and cousins lived close by, and Paul and Nathan especially loved playing with Peter and Tobey, my brother Jon's boys.

During the summer, before Nathan turned four, I took him and Paul to the first Star Wars movie. We went to the Drive-In Theater, and they sat in the front seats so they could see the movie better. It did not interest me at all, therefore I fell asleep in the back seat. When the lights came on, they woke me up, and I said, "OK, let's go!" But the kids quickly let me know that was just intermission (ugh!). This was the beginning of their love for Star Wars. Unsurprisingly, this first Star Wars movie turned out to be one of Nathan's earliest memories.

When Nathan was going to be four years old, I asked him what he wanted for his birthday. He said, "A surprise party!" I laughed at that request and set out to plan it. When the day arrived, we were still in Blue Hill. Hank took Nathan for a walk down to the park, while Jon and Sandy came over with their family. We all hid, and when Nathan walked in the front door, we jumped out and shouted, "Surprise!" He was so happy to see everyone there for his birthday. I had made his cake with a Star Wars figure on top. He loved everything about Star Wars and still does. He was so excited about the figure on top but he didn't care much about the cake.

Summer in Blue Hill was always special for my kids. In later years, they counted the days when school would be out so we could go to Gram's. One summer after he retired, my Dad put an above-ground swimming pool in the backyard. I guess he wasn't finding enough to keep busy because that pool more than consumed his time! It had a pump and a little step ladder for the kids to get into the water. Sometimes there would be five or six grandkids in the pool having a blast together. However, it was placed a little too close to the apple tree. Dad found himself constantly cleaning leaves out of the pool. Still, it was a wonderful investment for the time the kids used it, and Grampa was there with them.

I remember a time when the kids were older and their cousins were spending the day. Six kids sitting around bored, my mother wouldn't have it! She dreamed up a challenge for them. There would be three teams of two: Paul and Peter, Nathan and Tobey, and Corey and Becky. She gave each team an old sock that they had to plant at the top of the mountain. The first team home would get a prize. The base of the Blue Hill Mountain was about a mile from my parents' home, and the climb was a little less. The three teams all set out running, probably not for long on that hot summer day. Upon reaching home, they anxiously asked for the prize. Mom said there were popsicles in the freezer. Early arrivals acquired the privilege of choosing first. I think they were a little disappointed but they'd never show that to their grandmother. The lesson for them was that they can always find something fun to do whether there's a reward at the end or not. They all agreed the day was the prize!

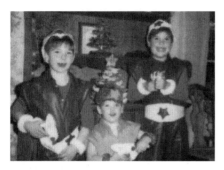

My mother did many other things for her grandchildren. She was a very creative person in many diverse ways. She made sets of stuffed animals of the Winnie the Pooh characters when my children were very small. One year when we arrived for the summer, she had totally papered a room in the house just for the kids. The wallpaper had a Disney theme, and she made quilts with Disney characters for the two beds. Mom loved having the kids around to do special things for, and they always loved being with her.

One Christmas when we happened to be home, my mother made special alien outfits for six children: our three boys and Jon's three kids. Becky, Jon's daughter, was the only girl (my Emily hadn't been born yet) and her outfit was a little skirt. She and Corey were about four and three at the time. The boys all had shirts, pants, and hats that made them look like they were from another planet. Mom used a silky green and yellow material with lots of silver sparkle in just the right places. Their hats had silver antennae that made them look like outer space aliens. She also bought each of them a toy laser gun, which of course made a noise. The kids were all delighted with their gifts and ran around the house making the gun noises. Of course, these outfits were their favorite gift. No need to open any more. Their Christmas was complete!

I haven't even mentioned Mom's fantastic cooking! Sometimes, waking up in the morning, you could smell the aroma of fresh donuts. It would draw you down to the kitchen where at 8 a.m., she'd already made a couple of pies, and oatmeal bread was rising on the counter. The donuts were warm and ready for anyone to help himself, an amazing treat for all of us! Growing up in this house as a child, I had taken these things for granted. As a young mother of three boys, I was able to more fully appreciate all she had done for us, and for others. It wasn't unusual for neighbors or friends to be in the neighborhood and just drop in for coffee and homemade donuts. In this town, my mothers' cooking was famous. She baked for all the food sales and church suppers, as well as helping my grandmother with her orders for goodies. The Blue Hill Public Library was across the road, and Mom's friends knew they were always welcome for a coffee and donut after visiting the library. Our home earned the name "Grand Central Station," especially when my brothers and I were teenagers, bringing our friends over for a visit or a meal.

As my boys grew older, we decided they needed more activity so we sent them to the Nichols Day Camp, which was actually in Sedgwick on Walkers Pond. They'd take their lunch and bathing suits and board the bus waiting at the school, at nine in the morning. At four in the afternoon they arrived home, tired campers. They had spent their day enjoying all the activities, including swimming, sailing, crafts, music and games of camp.

Another tradition that happened at least once each summer was a family meal, with my siblings and their children. My mother would cook up a storm, and we'd have something super delicious and top it off with pies for dessert. My dad loved pie, so she always had a seasonal pie for dessert, usually with a scoop of ice cream on top. We all loved to hear Dad's stories of his work or childhood. He wasn't much of a talker but he did know how to tell a good story, which usually ended in a lot of laughter.

Now my brothers and I and spouses continue this tradition our parents had started, by occasionally getting together for a meal. There are always stories to tell and usually some apple pie or dumplings to highlight the evening. We love to tell and retell stories of our childhood, as viewed through different eyes. We all have our own versions and argue over the details of the events. By the end of the evening the laughter gets so loud at least one spouse prefers to watch the news on TV. I feel bad for the spouses because sometimes it's hard to follow our silly stories!

The best part of the family dinner is the fact that it does continue to this day. Not often, maybe twice a year. But for that one evening, my brothers and I are kids again, reminding each other of days gone by that were filled with childhood joy!

CHAPTER TWELVE

THE PULL-THRU

It was the end of our vacation in Maine and we were headed back to Spruce Lane with a new piano in the U-Haul trailer behind our car. My goal was for the children to hear as much music in their environment as possible.

Nathan was about to turn one year old. Still he didn't walk. I told myself it was the colostomy bag that made him off balance. We had a round hassock in the living room that we sat Nathan on to take his Birthday Picture. We thought he was perfectly balanced on it, and he fell right forward landing on his nose. He cried. I felt so guilty, but the whole thing happened so fast it was almost comical. Consequently birthday pictures were all showing his red nose and not many smiles.

Dr. Eraklis had scheduled the "pull-thru" operation for a couple weeks after Nathan's first birthday. This meant the colon would be brought down to the point where his anal opening should have been. The surgeon would cut away the skin and the colon would be pulled through so bowel movements would be normal. Only, normal bowel movements were never to happen for Nathan because he had no sphincter muscle. His colon stopped growing high in his abdomen as he was developing in the womb. Therefore, the sphincter muscle, which is usually on the end of the colon and controls the bowel movement, was never there. The colostomy finally would be closed permanently and Nathan would be left with scar tissue in that area of his abdomen. We had been waiting for this day since he was born: just to be able to diaper him the usual way. Pampers had just appeared in the marketplace, and I was excited to try them out. However, this also would never be an option for Nathan.

Dr. Eraklis, at Boston Children's Hospital, did all of Nathan's surgeries at that facility, and became Nathan's primary doctor for those early years. Dr. Eraklis always explained things to me walking down the hall. "Walk with me," he'd say. Sometimes he would sit in a lobby or waiting room, and draw some pictures of what his plan was in the surgery, or just what Nathan looked like on the inside. He must have had an office but I never saw it.

It was extremely difficult for either of us to be with Nathan during a surgery because of Paul. The first two years of Nathan's life Paul was between two and four-years-old, so one of us needed to be with him. Hank knew of people who had been discharged from the service for having extreme problems at home. These problems were so intense and needed the support of the serviceman to the extent he missed too much work time. If this happened to us, we would lose the insurance, and without it things would have been very difficult for our family. So once again, Nathan was alone for this surgery and it was tearing me up inside. We talked to the doctor before and after the surgical procedure, as well as nurses throughout the week. One time when Nathan was hospitalized longer than a week, Hank took me to the hospital for a weekend while he stayed with Paul. Boston Children's Hospital provided a cot in the lounge area on Nathan's floor; equipped with a sheet, pillow, and blanket, as well as face cloth and toothbrush! They tried to help the parents as much as possible and certainly did make it very comfortable for us. Other parents were also spending the night in the same area while some mothers chose to put a blanket on the floor beside their baby's crib. It was very humbling to see their devotion.

I met many parents of very sick babies while visiting Nathan at different times. It appeared that many of these babies had conditions much, much worse than Nathan's. I always felt blessed that his surgeries would be over early in his life. (That was my expectation because of what I'd been told.) The nurses told me the babies with no parents around were the easiest for them to care for, and most content. One mother, who made it a habit to stay right by her child every waking moment, couldn't even leave to get a meal without the child wailing uncontrollably. She felt compelled to wait until the child was asleep. This routine for days on end must have been exhausting for her. She did tell me that in my absence, she would sometimes talk to Nathan while her baby slept. For that I was extremely grateful.

Hank and I were so excited that Nathan was finally going to be free of colostomy bags and dressings. At this time we thought he would be able to wear a diaper normally. The surgery was a huge success, Dr. Eraklis did an awesome job closing the colostomy. Nathan's skin healed on his abdomen very quickly.

It always surprised me at how rapidly he would heal after a surgery. By the time we brought him home, a week after surgery, his colostomy site was looking very good. The doctor had done such a good job stitching him up. But we now had a new problem, which was keeping the skin on his bottom from breaking down. Dr. Eraklis said, "Over time that skin will toughen up." I learned that air and water were two elements that would contribute greatly to healing. I also discovered putting Nathan down for a nap in a warm room with no diaper would help heal the skin.

But our big problem was figuring out how to keep that skin clean when his bowel seemed to be constantly emptying right over it. Finally out of frustration I called the hospital for help. They told us Nathan would need to have a bath every six hours around the clock. He must be soaking in the tub for a good fifteen minutes with each bath.

If that was what it would take, then we would do it! We started before Hank went to work, around six o'clock. I did the noon bath and Hank helped me after supper when we dressed Nathan all cuddly and warm in PJs ready for bed. Shortly after midnight, we were at it again. I tried to convince Hank to sleep because he had to get up early for work the next morning. I would be able to catch cat naps while the kids were napping. But he always got up with me every night. We put three or four inches of water in the tub and had a few toys for Nathan to play with. It didn't seem to bother him at all that we woke him up in the middle of the night. We made a routine of bath, a feeding time, and a little rocking before putting him back in the crib; then he would usually go right off to sleep.

This routine went on for a few weeks but we couldn't seem to get the bleeding under control; it wouldn't stop, and we were both exhausted. Very reluctantly we made the call to the hospital, and two physically and emotionally drained parents surrendered their child back to Boston Children's Hospital. The separation was painful for Hank and me, but it did allow us to get some much needed rest. We needed to be strong and healthy for our baby when we could bring him home again.

I learned that sometimes when parents are dealing with a child needing this much care, they forget what all the stress of that kind of everyday situation does to their own bodies. The focus is so much on your baby that when he does have to go back to the hospital, you finally realize how totally exhausted you actually were. Your mind is full of the guilt that you weren't able to care for your baby enough to keep him out of the hospital. And for me the guilt that I couldn't be with him there. This is when parents need to take a step back and trust the professionals to be able to do what we couldn't in a home situation.

My advice to the reader, if you happen to have a child that needs most of your time and attention, is to use that time when the professionals are caring for his needs to rejuvenate body and soul. Do the things you weren't able to when you were so focused on the care of your baby. Go shopping, or visit a friend. For me, it was putting more time into reading and doing activities with my older child. Maybe even sitting at my piano for a few minutes to feed my own soul.

Nathan was in the hospital about one week. I called every day to be sure he wasn't crying for us or miserable away from home. I just don't know what I would have done if they responded in the affirmative, but they didn't. The nurses always assured us he was an excellent patient to take care of and everyone's favorite. That sounded familiar, and it put my mind at ease. When we actually went to get him, Nathan was in great spirits and happy to come with us. He looked healthy and his skin was mostly healed. The struggle to maintain healthy skin on his bottom wasn't over, but for now we were encouraged and had new optimism for the task.

The next few months Nathan was hospitalized several times for this same reason: to heal that raw, bleeding skin. It was several years before that skin would become firm enough so it wouldn't break down constantly. It was impossible to keep him clean for any length of time, and diaper changes had to be done very often. There was a time when we had taken Nathan to the hospital for the skin to heal, and the doctor kept putting us off from bringing him home. It wasn't healing as fast this time as he or we had expected. I was very frustrated, not knowing when we could pick him up, when I received a picture in the mail from the hospital. One of the Hospital Auxiliary Ladies had taken a picture of Nathan lying on his stomach, in a long stroller bed, smiling at the camera. She had been taking him for a ride around the ward. To be able to see that smile really did make my day and I felt so grateful to that volunteer. Shortly after receiving the picture, the call came to pick Nathan up. I remember walking in to the ward and seeing him standing in a johnny, holding his Humpty Dumpty at the nurses' station. Happy were the days when we brought him home.

Nathan still had the ureterostomies at this time, so I couldn't use Pampers. They wouldn't go high enough on his abdomen to cover the draining openings. We were still using cloth diapers when we were at my mother's house, and she had bought me a pail with a handle and cover for the dirty diapers. We figured out a cleaning solution to soak the diapers in until I could wash them in the washing machine. Another idea she had was to put a liner in the diapers. We bought pastel-colored disposable dish cloths that were very soft. I cut them in rectangles that would fit in the diaper. This held the majority of the bowel movement and protected the diaper somewhat. They were easily discarded as well.

Little Nathan's personality really didn't reflect all he had been through or was presently experiencing. He would take everything as it came; maybe because he didn't know anything different. Nathan laughed and cried like any other child. He strove to keep up with his brother, as siblings do. The time it took for me to take care of his needs was just a bother to him, keeping him from playing with Paul. Paul was upset when we left Nathan in the hospital but we were able to convince him that his brother would be home again in a few days. These were the times Paul would stay with his friend, Jon, next door, while we took Nathan to and from Boston. It gave him a chance to play rather than to sit in a car for a long ride, which he really didn't like. Meanwhile Paul received a lot of "only child" attention throughout the days Nathan was hospitalized. He came to understand we were right, and his brother always did come home after a few days.

CHAPTER THIRTEEN

MORE SURGERY

Approximately six months after the pull-thru things were going well so Dr. Eraklis was ready to close the ureterostomies. We would take him to Boston Children's Hospital for the surgery. I still remember the feeling of my stomach churning as I left my baby at the hospital. It wouldn't stop until we brought him home. It was so hard giving him over to someone else's care when it was so critical. Throughout the times of surgery, I kept reminding myself that God loved him more than my heart would ever be capable of. And if God had the "whole world in His hands," I knew He had my baby in His hands as well. So I chose to trust Him for all Nathan would be going through. I thanked God for the surgeons and always prayed for them, as well as for Nathan.

The surgery, which was done on both ureterostomies, was only successful on one side. The opposite side still leaked urine. Everything was working for him to urinate normally, and still the one side had a leak. The doctor decided Nathan needed to heal and live with it this way for a while. When he was a little older, they'd go in again and close that leaky opening. Meanwhile, he would need a small tube for drainage to be put in that opening so the skin wouldn't grow over and cause the urine to back up into his kidneys.

At twenty months Nathan was able to move his body more easily and play like other children. To our relief, he had started walking around the age of eighteen months. With the exception of the drainage tube, his abdomen was feeling quite normal, for him. At the beginning of his life, Nathan's body must have felt very different from how most babies feel. But it was all he ever knew, so all these surgical changes must have felt different to him, even as we pronounced it normal. His transition times after the surgeries were so unnoticeable from his behavior. Nathan acted like he'd always been that way, as he adjusted almost immediately. When I think of the enormous change in his abdomen after the colostomy was closed, I would have expected some kind of reaction from him.

Presently, our big problem with this drainage tube was naptime and night time. He was rolling over a lot, which caused us to be concerned that the tube might get pushed up inside of him. The doctors assured me this couldn't happen. I often wondered if the doctor just didn't want me to worry about this, or if he really believed it couldn't happen. I certainly had no medical training, but it only seemed like common sense to me that if the baby rolled over on a tube, it could go in further and follow that ureter up to the kidney. This whole tube thing continued to make us uncomfortable, and we became very anxious for that final surgery to be done.

Usually naptimes were short enough and I watched closely to get him up immediately when he woke up. It was mornings that we almost always found the tube had come out and was lying on the crib sheet. Skin had already started growing over the opening: the example I had referenced earlier of a baby's skin healing too quickly. Just a few short hours at night were enough to make it totally heal so no urine could drain through. The doctor had told us that if this happened we'd have to forcibly poke through the skin to allow the urine to come out. We tried, but neither of us could bare the screams and Nathan fighting us. The only alternative was to take him to the dispensary on the base. Hank usually did this around six a.m. before work, where he and the PA on duty would manage to get the tube in again. I know for a fact that PA dreaded to see Hank bring Nathan in those many mornings! One of them would hold him on the table while the other pushed the tube through skin that had grown over the opening in the night. Blood and urine would gush through and Nathan would scream.

But as soon as the tube was in place and securely taped, he would settle down and be okay. It was a blessing for me when Hank was able to do that. If Hank had duty and I was home alone, he left the car and walked the train bridge, while I took Nathan and Paul, too, to the dispensary. In that case, the PA was very kind and used a nurse to take Hank's place. Paul liked to play in the waiting room with the toys he found there. Nathan was a brave little baby boy but it had to hurt and they would pass me a whimpering baby. My heart wanted to cry with him. This tube didn't fall out every night but there were quite a few times we made that early morning trip to the dispensary.

One morning when Nathan woke up, the tube was out and I couldn't find it. I looked on the sheets, under the crib, and all around on the floor. We kept the bedroom empty of anything but his crib, changing table, and bureau just in case something like this happened. Hank helped me look; it was nowhere to be found. What I was told would never happen, did. We took him to Boston Children's Hospital and an X-ray showed the tube had wrapped around Nathan's kidney. I was so angry and frustrated that this happened, and in my care. He shouldn't have had to go through this extra surgery! I was devastated about that because I always had a feeling it could happen, but nobody seemed to know how to stop it.

Nor would they admit that it could even happen in the first place!

Later that summer we saw a urologist who felt he needed to measure how much urine was coming from the leaky ureter. Nathan had to wear a plastic container bag strapped to the side of his leg, with a tube which came from the ureter to the bag. That year in Connecticut was the hottest summer I can ever remember. Day after day, without a break, the thermometer would reach 100+ degrees. You couldn't fit an air conditioner in the windows of our house because of the way they opened. The best we could do was to find a shady tree to sit under and pray for a breeze. We put a kids' wading pool under a shade tree in the front yard for them. Paul was eager to jump right in and splash. Because of all of Nathan's paraphernalia, we could only allow him to wade in the pool and splash water from the outside. Hank built a little chair just Nathan's size so he could sit close to the pool and splash his feet.

That miserably uncomfortable summer was bad for the whole family, but Nathan was the one wearing a plastic bag close to his skin throughout the heat wave. The days seemed to be endless and every day the same. Finally, the end of the summer brought a break in the extreme heat. Nathan could look forward to throwing that bag away after the surgery in early September. This time everything went well, and the leaky ureter was closed successfully. Now all of his plumbing was hooked up correctly and working. Happy Nathan! Happy family!

CHAPTER FOURTEEN

GENERATIONAL CHILDHOODS

Here I would like to pause to discuss the differences of my generation's childhood and my children's childhood. The way my three brothers and I were raised was very different from the way I raised my four children. Yet many things are the same like our basic morality and love of family.

The four Woodward children were lucky enough to grow up in a coastal town. My mother stayed at home with us until my youngest brother, Tom, was in school. After that she always had a job but she would try to take vacation during our school vacations, to be home with us. Otherwise there would be a list of instructions for each of us to follow. The rule in our house was chores before going anywhere. And when leaving the house or neighborhood a note had to be left on the chalk board, of where we were and when we'd be home. Mom also allowed us to call her at work if we needed to ask her permission to go somewhere. From a young age we were allowed to make those choices.

It must be mentioned here that my grandmother, my father's mother, lived downstairs in our house. She was very lame but also very independent. So my mother knew there was an adult around if we needed anything. My brothers and I loved spending time with Gram, mostly one on one. She enjoyed playing card games, and many evenings it was fun to have time playing cards alone with Gram.

The wonderful smells in Gram's kitchen drew us downstairs many times. We tried to find excuses to walk through hoping she'd have an extra cookie for us. She did cooking for organizations around town, like the yacht club or the country club. They ordered dozens of different kinds of cookies, bars and other goodies for their parties. Gram always had time for us kids, except those times when she was cooking and asked us to not run through her kitchen, which was our short cut to the barn. From her back kitchen door, we could go out on the porch and to the backyard and barn.

When we were young we liked to play in the barn on a rainy day. I could fill pages with what we found to do out there. My Dad had all kinds of interesting tools as well as lots of pieces of wood, old tires, boxes, etc. There was a ladder in the back of the barn that led to a loft (with lots of holes in it). I don't remember falling through but I do remember at one time or another each of us got a nail in our foot from that barn. "These are the things that make you tough," my parents used to say.

One of our favorite places to play was the Dodge Woods across the road from our house. My brothers built brush camps and trails through the woods. They built a lookout platform high in a tree with narrow boards nailed to the tree for a ladder. Nearby there was a very small camp that had two beds and a small stove in it, where I remember spending a night with one of my girlfriends when we were about eleven years old. It was cold but that little stove kept us warm and cozy. We did get in trouble with my brothers by melting crayons right on the stove top itself! The boys had gone to a lot of trouble to get that stove, and didn't appreciate the display of colored wax melted on the iron.

The majority of the tall trees were evergreens and smelled wonderful. As young people we loved playing in the woods and enjoying all the great smells, and sights. Before I leave the Dodge Woods, I must say there were the largest, reddest, juiciest wild raspberries growing right there in "our woods." In the summer heat you could smell the raspberries, and it was our favorite spot for picking.

Every year we anticipated picking berries with Mom. She would take her raspberries home and make a pie or muffins. Jon and I liked to pick them to sell to the local market. Tom and Sam were just trying to keep what they picked in their buckets! The raspberries were growing in and around briar patches. The test was to be able to not spill your bucket as you kept your balance walking on branches. Usually Tom and Sam would give up and eat what they'd picked but Jon and I looked forward to what we'd do with our berries: the reward at the end. After we sold them to the market, we'd take our money and go across the road, to the counter at the drug store and order a root beer float. It was usually a very hot summer day and we felt we earned the treat.

Sometimes we liked to go swimming at the Big Rock, if the tide was in. The Big Rock was about five minutes, by foot, from our house. All four of us would go, and we met many friends there. In recent years, that beach area is referred to as the Town Park and has been upgraded with a beautiful picnic area as well as playground. But during our childhood, it was referred to as the Big Rock by everyone in town. If the tide was high enough, we could run and jump off the back of the rock and sometimes even touch the bottom. It was a great way to spend a hot summer afternoon. As small children, we would check for the high tides and wait for Mom to get her chores done so she could walk us to the beach. Occasionally we'd stop on the way at Sally's Shop, and pick out a new pail and shovel. When we were in our teen years, we'd go with friends and Mom trusted us because we all could swim, even though she never wanted to learn herself.

Growing older we ventured further from home. The mountain beckoned and we couldn't resist the adventures waiting for us there. Dad had a woodlot on the backside of the mountain so he often took the boys up there with him, cutting and piling wood to bring home for the furnace. My three brothers also built a camp up there. When we were younger it was very rustic, but by the time they became teens they made it a very comfortable camp, and it gave them a place to get away on their own.

On long summer days when we couldn't think of something to do, we'd just climb the mountain. It was only 1,000 feet high and it had a fire tower on top. Up in the tower, a man with binoculars would be watching for fires around the whole area below, and would notify the firehouse if he spotted anything. On a good day the view was extremely beautiful; you could see for miles around.

My Dad loved to sail but my Mom did not like boats. When we were in high school Dad acquired a sail boat. He worked on that Brutal Beast until it was sea worthy. After giving my brothers a few basic instructions about sailing, and sending all of us to Coast Guard Safety Training, he allowed us to use it at will. Of course, there was no motor on it to help us in and out of the harbor. Blue Hill Harbor has a place called the Narrows, and when the tide turned, quite often there was no wind. Many nights my father would drive down to the yacht club and shine his headlights out towards the Narrows. Sometimes it would be a dead calm and you could hear the boys talking in the boat. Before we had the sailboat, Dad and Jon had built an outboard motor boat, so Dad took Jon's boat and towed the boys into the mooring. In my memory, this happened many times, either just as we were sitting down for supper, or much later in the evening.

My three brothers and some of their friends built a real Tom Sawyer raft. It was kept in a cove by what we called the Dynamite Rock. It was very rustic and the only paddle was a board. One afternoon my friend, Nancy, and I decided we'd take it for a test run. We both had our bathing suits on because we figured before the day was over, by choice or not, we'd be wet. With a little luck on our side we were able to maneuver it around the corner to the Big Rock swimming area. Just beyond the Big Rock was a small island, called John's Island, and we thought it would be fun to go out there. Besides the tide was in our favor: it was going our way! We easily got to the little island, and took turns going ashore, did some wading, and generally felt pretty proud of ourselves for being able to do all this so easily. When it was time to head back, a little breeze had come up and the tide was not in our favor. We struggled the rest of the afternoon trying to get back to the beach. Nightfall was imminent, and all the beach goers had left, but someone heard our cries for help. A very kind person took pity on us and came with a boat to tow us in to the beach. The next thing we knew there were several cars shining their headlights down across the bay towards us. We felt the whole town knew what we did, and when we arrived, Nancy and I hung our heads as we walked by the many well-wishers. We were exhausted from the long ordeal and totally embarrassed. I still remember how humiliated we felt.

In the winter, my three brothers and I would go sliding wherever we could find an adequate hill. One time we'd had a blizzard and school was cancelled, so we headed for the mountain and noticed the snow plow had not cleared the road in front of the mountain trail. At one point that road went down very steeply and it would give us a long ride, so we decided to slide there. On the way to the mountain we picked up a bunch of friends. About a dozen of us were up there sliding having the best time on that unplowed road, until the plow truck appeared. All of us defiantly lined up across the whole width of the road to stop the plow truck driver. We held our hands up to the truck driver and argued for him to come back later. Even after our magnificent display of solidarity, he wasn't taking orders from a bunch of hoodlums. The plow driver spoiled our sliding for that day! We went away grumbling and shaking our fists at the driver; but ultimately decided we'd just have to find another place, even if it was not as fun.

Other things the Woodward kids did in the winter were skating, building tunnels and forts, and having snowball fights with the kids on the other side of town. Our skating parties were at the Salt Pond, a long tidal pond, not even a mile from our house on Parker Point. A small bridge was situated between the pond and ocean. A large rock right at the pond's edge was perfect for putting skates on or building a bonfire. Usually someone brought an old tire and we'd have a large bonfire that lit up the ice and we could see for a long distance out. Weekend afternoons were often spent on the Salt Pond; but nights were the best. There were usually a lot of people on the pond, as long as the ice was clear.

Sometimes we'd play "crack the whip," making a long line of skaters skating together until the first person in line stopped suddenly, causing the others to go around him like a whip. It didn't take long before I learned not to be the last person in line.

I think the most profound difference between growing up in the 1950s and '60s rather than the 70s and 80s, or even today, is the safety factor. We always felt safe in this small town of 1500 people. Our parents never worried about things that could happen. I think they were too busy worrying if they would be able to pay the bills. They taught us, and then they trusted us. That doesn't mean that the ice couldn't have cracked and swallowed one of us up or that one of us couldn't have fallen out of the sailboat and drowned in the bay. But they never would discourage us from doing what we wanted, as long as it was somewhat reasonable. When I was growing up, young people were given serious responsibilities of all kinds at young ages. From the fifth grade on I was responsible for supper, cooking every night before my mother got home from the dentist office where she worked until six o'clock. She taught me to use the gas stove and trusted me with it. My brothers had to go down into the cellar and fill the wood furnace. Splitting wood to fill the wood-box was another of their responsibilities. They were taught to use chain saws and axes at young ages. Once we started grammar school, we were old enough to be left alone for short periods of time.

Today young people have chores and obligations but I don't think they are left unsupervised as much as we were, or given as much responsibility for family duties as we had. With TV, radio and internet, we hear more about bad things that happen and I think parents are very protective of their children. I know I was, and sometimes regret that my children didn't have the carefree childhood that my brothers and I were privileged to experience.

I will forever be grateful to have been raised in an extraordinarily beautiful coastal town in Maine, with the mountain and ocean so close together. Its' a picturesque environment for all who live, visit and grow up here. It was such a blessing to learn and grow in this setting, where people knew and cared about neighbors, especially families. Most importantly, I'm grateful to have had the parents that we did. Both of them were hard workers, dedicated to God and family, and raised four children with lots of love, trust, and support.

* * *

The four Fenders children had very different childhoods. They were children of the military housing phenomenon, for the most part. The youngest two, Corey and Emily, were not in military housing as much as the older two, Nathan and Paul. At every opportunity, we would bring the kids home to Blue Hill. I wanted them to see how carefree life could really be for them. It was a passion for all of them to have these summer days in Blue Hill to look forward to.

Living in so many different military housing areas, Paul and Nathan found it was fun to explore different playgrounds when they were small. Several places where we were stationed, there were a variety of playgrounds located in different spots around the housing area. The boys were still too young to go to a playground alone unless, of course, it was one of those that was located right behind our house and I could easily see them. In Cape May, the last duty station before coming back to Blue Hill to live, the boys all had bikes. They were old enough now to go off on their own. The housing area was large and open and they quickly learned their way around. They rode all around the housing area, on the base, and even further, if I knew where they'd be. Nathan and Corey enjoyed going on base to play tennis or run the obstacle course, set up for the men in "boot camp", when nobody was using it. The cool thing for them was to show their I.D. Cards to get on base; it felt like a big deal to a kid.

Because of Hank being in the military and all the moves to different duty stations, our kids had opportunities growing up that my brothers and I never had. We were able to take them to several different zoos . We took them on train rides, and we went to museums, not to mention just sight-seeing everywhere we lived. Paul and Nathan particularly enjoyed visiting Gillette Castle in Connecticut. During school vacation one year when we lived in Cape May, we took them to Washington D.C. We visited the Smithsonian Museum, The Air and Space Museum, the Lincoln Memorial, as well as some of the government buildings.

In Cape May, Hank would take the kids to the Wildwood Boardwalk to go on rides and enjoy the amusements there. On special occasions he would take the boys out for a night to see the World Wide Wrestling Federation(WWWF). All three of the boys really enjoyed that event while Emily and I stayed home for a girls night in. Another time I took her on a bus trip to Philadelphia for a Disney on Ice Show.

When we lived in Charleston, Paul was about four years old and Nathan was two and a half. We thought we were closer to Disney World than we'd probably ever be again so we took the two boys. Paul loved it and had pictures taken with all the characters, but Nathan was frightened of the people in costume, so I had to hold him while Hank took the picture. We were able to find rides and things Nathan would enjoy even at such a young age, so it turned out to be a good time for all of us. Nathan recalls that he actually remembered the Dumbo Ride, even at that early age. Later, when we were living in Cape May, we took another trip to Disney World. Emily

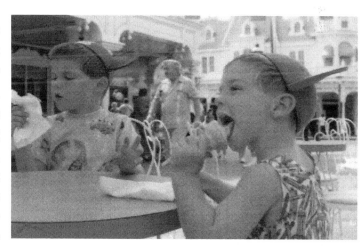

was four, Corey was ten, and Paul and Nate were in their teens. Similar to the first time we all had a wonderful experience. This time the teenagers were allowed to go off by themselves. I think they liked that independence from the rest of the family. In contrast to the first visit to Disney World, there were many more things to see and do. Crossing the New Jersey State line on the way home, Hank said "Who wants to turn around and go back to Disney World?" Four voices from the back seat were cheering for that! Only one voice in the front seat was too exhausted to even think of it. I think he expected them to be so tired of riding in the car that they'd just be anxious to get home, like me.

One summer when we were living in Blue Hill, Nathan wanted to enter a race of dirt bikes going up the mountain. He didn't have the right kind of bike but Uncle Ron did, and allowed him to use it. Uncle Ron was my cousin's husband, a teacher at the high school, and a counselor at the day camp the kids attended. All the kids at camp called him Uncle Ron. Nathan did the race with that bike, which came back in a little different shape than when he left with it. (I believe the wheel was broken.) He was surprised when he came home with a trophy!

My boys loved the mountain just as my brothers and I did, and spent many summer days hiking up different trails to the top. There were wild blueberries growing in a field near the top if they needed a snack. It was always a good option for a long summer day when you didn't quite know what to do with your time.

When the boys were pre junior high and Hank wasn't around, I had my hands full with unruly kids and needed some help. One time the punishment for whatever Paul and Nathan had done (probably fighting with each other) was a day of work on Uncle Ron's farm. You could be sure he would need help haying in the summer. He brought the boys home and said that they were good workers. Another time when Corey was in high school he was out a little too late without calling us. His punishment was to get up early the next morning and pick green beans from a neighbor's garden. My friend had offered us all the beans we wanted and, since I planned to can them, this would be helpful. Corey grumbled, but he did it.

Each one of my children experienced Scouting. Hank and I had a Cub Scout Den for Corey and his friends in Cape May, and

I did Emily's Girl Scout troop throughout her grammar school years. Earlier, when we lived in Blue Hill for the two years before Emily was born, I did Cub Scouts with Nathan and Paul's age group. There always were plenty of kids that wanted to do scouting, 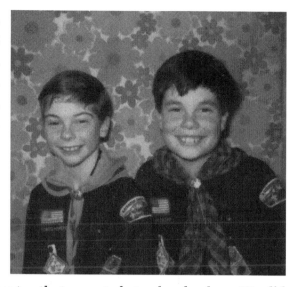 and never enough parents that wanted to be leaders. We did the parades, camping, cookies – the whole scouting experience. Paul was a Boy Scout when we lived in Blue Hill. His scout troop was having a kite contest at the Fairgrounds. Paul's grandfather helped him build a huge kite and then went to the Fairgrounds with him the day of the contest. They had a good time building it, but that day the wind wasn't cooperating and it was too hard to get a kite that large up in the air. The time together for grandpa and grandson gave the project significance.

In 1986, we were home for a summer vacation. Emily was three, and Hank decided to take her for a walk downtown. He went by a real estate office and noticed a camp for sale on nearby Toddy Pond. He did some research and we visited the camp and unanimously decided to buy it. The kids were all thrilled about it, and this camp turned out to be a terrific family investment. The camp was on the shallow end of the pond, so the kids were able to walk way out in the middle of the pond and still be able to touch bottom. I felt they would be safe out there, and they loved being on the water! All of them improved their swimming skills out on Toddy Pond. We spent many summer days at our camp, although it had no electricity and only an outhouse for a bathroom. But we had a gas refrigerator, gas lights, and a gas grill to cook on. Many happy days were spent swimming, boating and fishing at our camp. We even had some blueberry bushes in front of the camp.

My uncle gave us a row boat he wasn't using, to have at camp for the kids. Eventually we added a canoe and a couple of kayaks. The boys liked to paddle down the pond to a sandy beach when they were teens. As they became more proficient at swimming, they wanted to find the deeper water. As long as they were together and had some life jackets, we let them explore the pond's shoreline.

Many cook-outs and picnics took place at the camp with our extended family and friends. Several summers, before Paul and Nate had summer jobs, we spent most days at camp, where there was plenty for them to do. We bought a huge inflatable raft for them to take out in the middle of the pond and jump off. They had to go a ways out to find deep water for jumping. The boys and their cousins liked to play "King of the Raft." Because we were at the lower end of the pond, we didn't have much boat traffic, and I always felt safe with the kids in the middle of the waterway.

Directly in front of the camp was a small

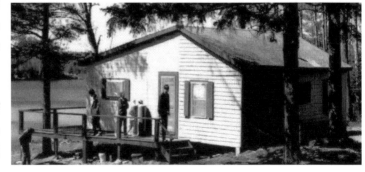

98

island. Everyone liked to paddle the canoe around the island which had lots of pond lilies on the other side. It was also very shallow, so it was a challenge to maneuver around the rocks without hitting them. Paul used it to practice swimming laps from the camp to the island and back. He was on the swim team in high school, so it gave him extra practice in the summer.

There were so many other adventures in their childhoods that I can't begin to remember them all. In comparing their childhoods with my generation, I'm convinced it is the safety factor that is the difference. The majority of my children's childhoods were supervised, whereas my brothers and my childhood had less parental involvement. Not that my parents didn't know where we were or what we were doing; they just weren't present as we were doing it most of the time. Without ever stating it or consciously thinking it, I believe they taught us and then trusted us. For the most part, we were trustworthy kids, although there were times when we'd get ourselves into trouble. I probably could write a chapter for each of us about our indiscretions; we definitely were not perfect!

But this is not to say my parents didn't do things with us. We had a family camping trip to look forward to every Labor Day. Dad would pick some remote area in northern or western Maine. Always, it would be on a lake, so we could go canoeing. I know, if my Dad had been alive when we bought the camp, he would have loved it. The only vacations Dad ever had was camping, because that was about all people could afford for vacations in those days. When Dad retired, he and Mom came to visit Hank and me in Hawaii. It was their first real vacation, and they spent three weeks with us and then went to visit my brother, Sam, in Oregon for three weeks. Dad talked about that vacation for years.

My kids had many opportunities for different kinds of vacations. Paul wasn't too impressed with his Boy Scout winter camping vacation experience. He said they went to sleep in a cabin that had snow in the corner. It didn't sound very appealing, although they did have a big fireplace in that cabin. And then there was the time Uncle Sam took him and his cousin, Peter, hiking. Sam liked to hike where there wasn't any path, so they had to cut the bushes as they went. Paul said he was slapped in the face by a bush more than a few times. It totally cured him of outdoor camping desires. Paul and Nathan did have vacations with their Youth Group in New Jersey. The annual ski trip in the Poconos was special for them to look forward to every February vacation. Also, in the summer, if we weren't in Maine, there were plenty of things to do on Cape May Beach and Boardwalk.

The topic of trust needs to be addressed about my children. As my parents trusted my brothers and me, I also trusted my children. We were all strong believers of "trust but verify", as our former President Reagan promoted. I tried to give them responsibilities as much as possible. Nathan was a good babysitter at a young age, and did that for other families in our military housing, as well as for a family when we lived in Blue Hill. Nathan and Paul both worked at the local grocery store. Emily and Corey also had jobs by junior high years. They may have been jobs that my brother, Jon, came up with for his construction business. Other things the kids did for jobs were camp counselors, babysitters, and blueberry raking, and Emily was a junior helper at a daycare. Corey worked with a landscaper who lived down the road from us. All of them paid, or earned scholarships, for the major part of their college educations. I guess, any lack of trust I felt in raising my children was towards society. It seems in my childhood, society in general was kinder and gentler and caused people to feel safer. In contrast during my children's childhoods with so much media, we were constantly hearing of kidnappings and other horrible things that would cause parents concern. As parents we became more vigilant.

In conclusion, I will just say that my childhood was very different from what my children experienced. In retrospect I can see many wonderful experiences that my children had because of being military kids, as well as the awesome childhood I was fortunate to have growing up on the coast of Maine. There's really no comparison: they were just different, and I'm thankful for all of them.

CHAPTER FIFTEEN

CHARLESTON

Our furniture was already in Charleston from our move from Groton, CT. Hank had to go to a Navy school in San Diego, so the family spent time in Maine waiting for him. It was hard for him to be away from the family at Christmas but even more troublesome when the Navy tried a last minute switch. With only two weeks to go before finishing school, Hank learned that the Navy changed his orders from Charleston, South Carolina to Norfolk, Virginia. We had everything set (household goods, housing list) for Charleston but now it would be total turmoil to reset for Virginia. With the help of the Senior Enlisted Advisor making a few phone calls, Hank was able to have his orders changed back to Charleston. It seems that the Navy was playing politics as the ship in Norfolk was about to leave for a six month deployment and the Charleston ship was returning and headed for the shipyard. He was tops in his class at the school in San Diego, which gave him a little edge when he spoke his request.

It was a long ride to South Carolina from Maine with two kids, two and a half and four years old. There were lots of stops and breaks, but we finally arrived in eighty-six degree temperatures! It was a treat for us coming south into this lovely climate, after the cold New England weather. Reaching Charleston, we had no place to stay since our military housing was not yet available. We spent the night in a hotel and made an appointment with a broker for the very next day. After a breakfast of Dunkin' Donuts, we were off with the broker to find temporary living quarters.

The first place he took us was a trailer park, which had a laundromat within walking distance, a very important commodity. The trailer was clean and pleasant and located near the base, so we took it. We had never lived in a trailer, so it was definitely a new experience. The two bedrooms were on opposite ends of the trailer, which made me a little uneasy because the kids were so far away from us. It took two months before housing became available, which seemed like a long time because there wasn't much for the kids to do. Very little of our own things came with us on our journey from Maine. The kids had a few toys, but there was no playground close by, so they played in the dust around the trailer with their trucks. Needless to say, they took many baths while we were living in that location. Some days Hank was able to get off work early, and we would take the boys exploring this beautiful area which was to be our home.

Because we only had one car and Hank needed it to go to work, the boys and I would take walks around the trailer park area. I met a lady in a nearby trailer who was most anxious to lend me books to read from her Harlequin Collection. She was worried I'd be too bored with no car to go anywhere. I was grateful for her kindness. It stayed pretty hot the whole time we were in Charleston. Thankfully, when we eventually moved into military housing, there was air conditioning. They provide us with a lovely single-story three bedroom duplex. Normally, if you have two children the same gender, you would get a two bedroom place, but because of Nathan's problems we were given the three bedrooms. Just outside the kitchen door was a carport, and behind that was a big storage room. We used the storage room for a playroom which had a door directly into the living room. The lay out of the house and yard was so convenient for a family with small children.

Situated behind all of the houses was a large community playground which everyone used. We felt very safe with the kids playing there as all of the mothers could see them from their windows. My boys loved playing with the neighborhood kids, especially the two girls who lived next door to us. Cindy was Paul's age and Michele was Nathan's age, and they played almost every day. Our house was on the corner and had a larger lot with a large shade tree. During the warm summer days as many as eight or ten neighbor kids would come to play under the tree with my kids. I joked about having my own daycare, and always had plenty of drinks for everyone. In those days the kids would play with trucks and cars under the trees. It was in the eighties all of January and continued to be very warm the whole time we lived there, so wintertime felt like summer to us.

My Mom came to visit in April, and we took her and the boys for a picnic at a park where the trees were beautifully draped with moss. Since we all came from the north, we never saw this type of tree. While we were there near a large lagoon, Hank and I wanted to take a canoe ride. Mom wasn't fond of being on the water in a small boat, so offered to stay behind with Nathan, who also declined the canoe ride. Paul, Hank, and I went and had a beautiful time. Hank took some pictures, and I watched diligently for any snakes that might surprise us in the water.

Charleston was so friendly compared to the cold atmosphere of Connecticut, where we had arrived in January a couple of years earlier. In the north, people were just trying to stay warm in their own homes and didn't much notice when new neighbors moved in. However, Charleston was much friendlier, and before our moving van was emptied we had neighbors from all around housing come to welcome us. Never before had I felt so welcomed! My next door neighbor, Marie, became my very best friend in Charleston. She was the mom of the two little girls that my boys liked to play with. The kids would watch a superhero show on TV, and we'd put towels on their backs, and they would pretend to fly around like Superman. Playing super-heroes became their favorite game.

Later in the summer, Marie pulled out her swimming pool for the kids and, while we were sitting there talking, we suddenly noticed her daughter, Cindy, and Paul were both swimming under water in eighteen inches of water! Seeing them swimming without any formal instruction really surprised both of us. They had taught themselves and were having the best time!

Paul loved to collect little bright green tree frogs that would suction their feet to our windows. Eventually they'd fall off and die and become stiff. He'd pick them up and put them in his pockets. Once we took a trip to Myrtle Beach, and when Hank took Paul out of the car, all these little frogs fell out of his pockets. It was the first time we realized he had a collection.

Nathan's third birthday came while we were in Charleston. We decided to invite about a dozen neighborhood kids and parents, because these were the friends my kids played with regularly. We set up the tables in our carport so everyone could be in the shade. Nathan's cake was a train, and each car was carrying a different kind of candy. The kids didn't seem to mind when the heat of the day melted the frosting. They were happy getting into the candy and ice cream, which tasted especially good on a hot day. In the air-conditioned house, Hank made balloon animals

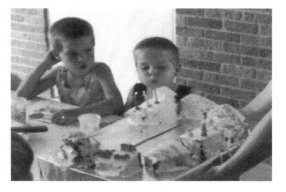

for each of the kids. They chose the colors of balloons they wanted. Everyone seemed to have a good time. The heat never bothered kids having fun together, but if they got too hot we all were thankful for the air conditioning inside.

All our memories about Charleston were happy for all of us, except Hank. Hank was still in the Navy, on the *USS Bowen,* and there were several things he was not happy about. He was extremely stressed at work because the Command was poorly organized. Hank was stationed on a ship that was in dry dock. He had to stand duty every six days, which was hard for me. At this time, Hank was a First Class Sonar Systems Tech, one of the top technicians on the ship. He was senior enlisted at the time but felt treated like a seaman recruit. Hank let his superiors know he wasn't very happy with their attitude, and showed them by getting out of the Navy and joining the Coast Guard, which he has never regretted. The Navy Executive Officer threatened Hank that they would give him a reenlistment code that would prevent him from enlisting in another branch of the service. They told him the Coast Guard would never take him and that he would have to re-enlist in the Navy. Little did they know Hank had already gone to see a Legal Officer in the Navy who said "no problem." Immediately Hank retired from the Navy, after eight years, and signed up for the Coast Guard. His rank and pay grade stayed the same but he was now an Electronics Technician. We were pretty excited thinking about the transition into the Coast Guard. Hank was excited to put the Navy behind and look forward to a new branch of the service. All I could think about was getting closer to Maine. I knew there were Coast Guard Stations in Maine!

The call from the detailer, who would tell us where Hank would be stationed, came one day when Hank was at work. I was so surprised, first because a detailer never calls a wife, and second because he said, "You'll be going to Governor's Island, New York." My response was, "You must be mistaken! We want to go to Maine; we don't even know where Governor's Island is!" He laughed and said, "Everyone in the Coast Guard goes to Governor's Island first." We'd been here only eight short months, and now we'd have to leave this beautiful place with all the friendly people, especially our dear neighbors. No more barbeques with our friends next door; no more super hero kids running from yard to yard to playground. I dreaded telling the boys, as my own heart was breaking. Marie and I had become very close, like sisters. We both loved to sew and went shopping for material together on weekends. Each week we made clothes for our kids and compared projects. I would definitely miss her. The boys wouldn't know how to get through a day without their little friends next door. It was heart- wrenching for all of us, with the possible exception of Hank.

Just before we heard from the detailer about our next destination, I had seen an ad in a paper for a piano teacher. A music store in a shopping mall that sold pianos also had their own teachers. One of my dreams was to teach piano all day, just have lessons, one after another. Hank said, "Why not try?" So we went to the store for the audition and interview. I was so excited at the possibility of being able to do my dream job, even for one or two days a week. It was right after that, before they could even call me to tell me whether I was chosen for the job, that we got the call to leave. I had to decline almost before they could offer me the job. This type of thing probably happens to military families often. Many families we've known of, had to change duty stations with only a few short weeks of notice.

My friend, who lived down the road from us in housing, offered for us to spend our last night with them. After the van was packed and the cleaning of the house was done, we headed to our neighbor's house. Three-year-old Nathan, holding my hand, was looking back crying, "I want to go home." We spent only a few months in Charleston but it sure did feel like home to all of us.

The cushion in our many moves was Maine. My parent's home was always open for us, especially between moves. We would go there until Hank got settled and got an apartment for us on Governor's Island. It turned out that I stayed in Blue Hill with the kids all fall, and after Christmas we finally moved into an apartment on Governor's Island. My parents never seemed to object to us staying with them for months at a time. That fall, I put Paul into a pre-K program a few days a week, to give him something special to do. Nathan attended a pre-school music activity a couple times a week. The movement helped his coordination, and he loved the music.

The stability that my parents' home gave our family was treasured by all of us. My parents continually received us with open arms and welcomed us for the duration of the time needed. The kids delighted in the time spent with their grandparents. Each time, after being home for several months, on the day we left Mom and Dad would stand on the front steps and wave. There was silence in the car for a long time, and I knew the boys were as sad as I was to leave. My childhood home was beginning to feel like home -away-from-home for my kids. They were just beginning to understand the impact that military life had on them. Friends were being left behind, and they were old enough to realize what that really meant to our family.

CHAPTER SIXTEEN

GOVERNOR'S ISLAND

Hank had to leave Maine the Monday after Thanksgiving to fly to Columbia, South Carolina to enlist in the Coast Guard. Following the enlisting he had to fly to Governor's Island, New York for his first Coast Guard assignment. It was a long day that ended in a city he was unfamiliar with. It was hard finding directions from the airport to the island without taking a taxi, which would have been very expensive on our tight budget.

Governor's Island was a Coast Guard Base off the tip of Manhattan. Hank had to get adjusted to being in the Coast Guard as well as to the new base. He arrived at work with no uniforms, so the officers wondered who he was. The problem was they had tops but no bottoms for his dress uniforms, and bottoms but no tops for his work uniforms. Eventually this was resolved and everyone knew he belonged there.

While living in the barracks temporarily Hank managed to get many things done. Getting assigned to an apartment was difficult as the Housing Office was closed-mouthed about what was available. One of Hank's fellow instructors at the training center told him that if the storage units on the first floor were empty and unlocked, it would indicate that the apartment was empty. His friend suggested we try to get into one of the high–rise buildings because it had air conditioning. One day he gave Hank a list of empty storage units, and Hank took it to the Housing Office. They were a little surprised at how he got that list, but Hank said it was common knowledge that you could see the storage units that were empty and then know the apartment was also free. They still tried to give him a building with no air conditioning but when he told them we had a piano and this particular building had a service elevator, that sealed the deal!

Another obstacle for Hank was trying to get paid before Christmas. He had hand delivered his pay sheet from the Navy. Payday was the fifteenth and thirtieth of each month. No paycheck was available on the fifteenth so Hank went to the pay office to find the problem. He was told they didn't have time to go through his Navy record because of the coming holiday and end of year tax reporting. Hank, knowing the system and who to talk to, was able to have a check issued in time for Christmas.

Governor's Island had a whole different feeling from the neighborhood in Charleston we'd left behind. The housing office finally assigned us an apartment in the high – rise building with air conditioning. " 877" was our building and there were several others with names just as charming! Our address was 5th floor, which was the button to push on the elevator. However when you get off the elevator you are actually ten floors up! Each apartment had an upstairs that added another floor. Although we were used to having a whole house, the apartment was very comfortable for the four of us.

New York was a totally unique way of living, unlike Charleston had been, or even Blue Hill. This really was city living, with these high-rise apartment buildings and so many people in a small space.

The island wasn't very large; you could easily walk the perimeter in a few hours. In our past military housing experiences, we'd been accustomed to much more freedom. The only driving for me would be to the commissary or exchange right here on the island. Across the river to Manhattan, we would find the subway or just walk through the city. Life on this island would take getting used to.

When we arrived on Governor's Island I was five months pregnant with our third son. Hank had been there when the movers arrived with our furniture, and he managed to get the apartment all set up and ready for us. He also found OB doctors for me in Greenwich Village, and managed to get time off to go with me on the subway for every appointment.

I was so depressed when we first arrived on Governor's Island, it felt like there was no way I'd ever be happy again. Hank would kiss me good-by in the morning before he went to work. One morning he said, "It's not that bad, is it?" With tears rolling down my face, I answered, "It's worse!" The contrast with Charleston was almost unbearable. I began to feel a similarity to the loneliness of Connecticut in the winter. There, everyone stayed in their own homes, and you had to really try to meet people and make friends. Here, there were hundreds of people living in close quarters, yet still that feeling of isolation overcame my whole being. I was so terribly unhappy that it took extra effort to keep the kids from noticing and reflecting my unhappiness. So I got my courage up and took my boys next door to introduce ourselves to the neighbor. She peeked out the door as if she were afraid we were selling something! After introducing the kids and myself as new neighbors next door, she let me know she was not interested. Our neighbor said she was getting ready to move within the next few weeks and was sorry she didn't have time or interest in meeting new people. So that door shut in our faces.

In spite of all that, inside our apartment was very pleasant. We had a million-dollar view of the Hudson River and the Statue of Liberty. We were able to watch boats and big ships that needed help from tugboats, out our picture window in the living room. On special occasions, the tugboats would spray colored water. The kids would watch for those particular occasions but otherwise were indifferent to the view.

There was a kitchen off the living room and a small bathroom downstairs. Upstairs there was a master bedroom and two very small bedrooms and a full bath. I could stand in my bedroom and look out at the playground in back of the building, ten floors below. The children on the playground, looked like tiny toys without distinguishable features. My children would never be able to go play without me, like they had in Charleston.

The laundry had to be taken to the basement laundromat located across from the storage units. I once figured there must be 600–700 people in our building and only one laundromat with about thirty machines and a few less dryers. The first few times I headed down the elevator with my laundry and two little boys was a disaster. There were so many people there, we couldn't find an empty machine. I discovered that certain cultures actually wash every part of their bedding from mattress pad to bedspread every week! These people would take six to eight machines at a time. My choice was to sit around and wait for a free machine or head back up the elevator dragging a basket of laundry and two unhappy little boys. At this time I was pregnant with my third son and feeling exhausted most of the time.   If I decided to wait, the boys would want to go out to that playground where I saw the "tiny people" from my bedroom window. The kids liked that, but because so many people lived in our building it was usually crowded.   Sometimes older children would be there and they would be a little too rough for my preschoolers to be around. So I had to watch them very closely.

Shopping turned out to be another hard thing for high – rise living. I noticed other people using wire carts to put their groceries in. We decided that would be easier than carrying bags separately, so we bought one. It became a much more efficient way to transport all our groceries in the cart in one elevator trip. I always hated elevators because of the possibility of getting stuck, so would take the stairs whenever there was a choice. Here there was no option but to use the elevators like the hundreds of other people who lived in this building. The alternative was a few too many stairs for a pregnant person.

When we first arrived they had fire drills and we were told everyone must evacuate the building but don't use the elevators. The first one came when I had just stepped out of the shower. So after wrapping my hair in a towel, putting on a robe and slippers, and gathering Paul and Nathan, we started down those endless flights. We met a few people along the way, and when we got outside there were only about twenty-five or so people. Obviously we were all the newbees! I asked the security guard if it was a joke or what? He responded with a shrug. Thankfully the elevators were available for our trip back up. We took part in the next few drills and then learned to ignore them like everyone else.

Governor's Island was a community within itself. The Island had its own school, church, commissary, exchange, bowling alley, and dispensary. There was even a fort. Some officers lived in the houses in the fort, where it was always fun to take a walk. The whole island was Coast Guard, and in order to take the ferry to the island you had to show your Coast Guard ID card. I felt very secure and safe on the island because everyone there either lived or had a job there, and mostly both. A bus would take people around the island if they needed a ride.

Many choices for playgrounds were available to us, consequently the kids liked trying different ones where they could have a variety of objects to play on. Occasionally I would meet other parents and we'd talk. It always seemed to be small talk about the island or the weather. Maybe it was the pace of the region that felt different to me. In Charleston, people took time to sit and visit with you and be neighborly. In New York, there seemed to be very busy people, always in a hurry. Even on the island, where we appeared to be an oasis from the city, there was a feeling of that busyness. Our actual living quarters with so many people close together, may have contributed to that feeling.

It took a long time before I finally met someone who could be a friend. In all my unhappiness, I decided to pray. I prayed God would send a friend for Paul, someone his age, so he'd have a companion when he started kindergarten. The apartment next door was empty and it wouldn't be long before a family would move in. The prayer was answered with more than I could have hoped for. The family was the same size as my family, and each child was the same age as my children. The mother was my age and eventually became my very best friend for the rest of the time we were there. Realizing the blessing was: if we just ask, God wants to bless us even more!

Pam and I found we had a lot in common besides our children. We both enjoyed walking early in the morning before the family was up. We took long walks around the island, shared recipes, went to ceramics classes together, and visited back and forth nearly every day. We even shared the Gospel because Pam was a new Christian and we both had a lot to learn about the Bible. Living right next door to each other made it easy to watch each other's kids as well. Pam was the exact kind of friend I needed to combat the loneliness eating at me when we first arrived on Governor's Island.

The laundry was one of my greatest frustrations, so I decided to pray for washing machines. Sometimes forgetting to pray early enough, God cleared the laundry room anyway! I never prayed when it wasn't answered with just the number of machines needed. I found out God loves us and cares about the little everyday things in our lives.

About four a.m. on May 29th we had to call for the island ambulance. Our third son was on the way. The ambulance driver decided to take a short cut on the other side of the river that took us over cobble stone roads. I tried to assure them everything was fine and they didn't need to hurry, but they continued to speed down the bumpy roads. Those rough roads may have contributed to a shorter labor because Corey was born at eight o'clock that morning. What a beautiful joy that was! I had been given gas right after he was born and came to just as Hank was wheeling him by. I said, "What's happening, that's Paul!" He weighed the same and looked the same as Paul – or was it the gas? I don't know, but Corey did grow into his own adorable looks and personality.

My mother had taken a vacation the week Corey was due. She was with us for the whole week before he decided to come. She only had time for a quick glimpse of him when Hank brought her to St. Vincent's Hospital, on the way to dropping her off at the airport. Mom's vacation time was gone so fast!

Now we had a brand new baby boy that we all adored. Corey was such a good baby and his brothers loved holding him and entertaining him. He watched them intently, and as he grew older followed them. He was such a happy baby. Everything was getting better for us as we learned the routine of living on this island. Daily life had a feeling of normal again. Not Charleston-normal but New York-normal now.

*   *   *

Nathan remembers my father coming to New York to visit us for a week without my mother. Dad took Paul and Nathan to visit the Statue of Liberty. It was around Christmas time, and Dad had a great time shopping by himself in New York City. He bought gifts for my family and a special ring for my mother. After thirty-five years of marriage and never having received an engagement ring, she finally was the happy recipient of a beautiful ring.

Lester, a young man who worked with Hank, turned out to be a great babysitter for my boys. Nathan said they loved to see Lester coming because he would play with them. Hank and I seldom left the kids, but occasionally we would obtain some theater tickets.

Hank was able to get tickets to take Nathan and Paul to a play up in the city. Nathan's memory of the Broadway play, Annie, was of the little girls jumping on the beds. He was especially impressed with that scene since it would never be allowed in our house. Five-year-old Nathan thought it looked like great fun!

Nate & Corey

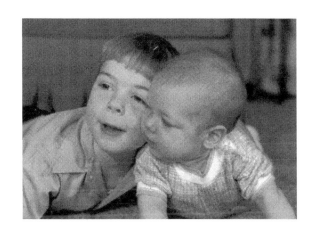

CHAPTER SEVENTEEN

ENEMAS AND TEARS

Nathan was four-years-old and I was getting nervous about his future in kindergarten. He was a year old when the surgeons did the break-through operation(often called the pull thru). Since that time it had been a challenge to keep his skin clear. We tried a variety of things to help him with the control of his bowel. Certain foods were helpful to him but others weren't. Corn was one thing he was never able to have; nor did he ever really miss it. I questioned every health professional we met. Finally we met a young doctor who was trying new things to help children with VACTERL association.

The doctor wanted us to try a routine of fleet enemas every other day. At the same time Nathan would be on a very low dose of opium. The combination was meant to totally clean him out in the morning and leave him clean all day. It sounded wonderful to me, and I was ready to try anything to help him be more comfortable and keep me out of the laundry room. Corey was an infant and sometimes would fuss for me when I was busy with Nathan. Paul was a great help and played with Corey downstairs or upstairs in his bedroom, singing, or making faces at him and making him laugh. Paul had a lot of experience doing that with baby Nathan, when he was little.

The fleet enema was about six ounces of fluid. I made a bed of towels on the bathroom floor and, at first, Nathan was very cooperative. I kept telling him it would be over soon and he could play. But it was very uncomfortable for him, plus something disagreeable that kept him from playing with his brother or watching cartoons. At first try he cried out because it may have been too cold, so we warmed it up just a little, which seemed to help. Sometimes Hank would dispense the enema but usually he would have to go to work before we were ready to do this.

Knowing it was going to be unpleasant each time, Nathan started dreading it and so did I. No matter how hard he tried not to cry there were always tears (for both of us). After administering the enema Nathan just stayed calm for a few minutes. Later I would push a hamper in front of him, while he was on the toilet, so he could play with his toys. That helped him to relax and enjoy himself playing, so the time passed easier. After about an hour he was ready to get dressed and start his day. This was a routine we carried on for months. Nathan had that enema every other day unless I decided he needed another day off.

At this time Nathan and I learned to pray together. We got everything ready and he was in position on the towels, and as I administered the enema we prayed that God would help us get through this easily and quickly. We prayed it wouldn't be painful and that Nathan would have a fun day after it was over. We prayed the weather would be good enough so we could go to a playground, where he loved to play. It always seemed he became more calm and peaceful as we prayed and thought of what we would do when this was over.

He was encouraged to take part in the prayers as much as possible. I wanted him to know God loves him even as we go through hard times. I wish I could say the enemas worked and he had a wonderful day of no soiling of clothing. These days were very trying for both of us, dealing with the frustration of no bowel control. However, the enemas didn't really produce the results we had hoped for.

The following summer when we were in Maine, Paul and Nathan cajoled me into taking them to the Drive-In Theater to see the first Star Wars movie. I was totally bored and remember falling asleep in the back seat of the car while the boys were in the front watching the movie. The kids just loved that particular movie. It became their favorite and whenever future Star Wars movies came out they would beg to go. Soon we started buying Star Wars figures for them to play with, and Nathan's favorite turned out to be anything Star Wars! So now when I pulled the hamper in front of him, after the enema routine, he played with his Star Wars figures.

My Dad was a carpenter for AB Herrick & Son, in downtown Blue Hill. One day he brought home a box full of beautifully smoothed and shaped wooden blocks that he had made for the kids. At other times he would bring home a refrigerator box and cut out the doors and windows for a playhouse for them. He built "brush camps" and turned his backyard into a playground with a swing set, sandbox, and swimming pool. Grampa definitely made my boys feel special when they came to Blue Hill. In New York, they didn't have the opportunity to run out the back door and have their own playground right there. Corey was an infant that summer, so he spent a lot of time sleeping. Sometimes I'd bring him out with us to nap. I liked being out in the backyard with the kids. It was a chance for me to be in a recliner lawn chair and get some fresh air myself. Mom was an awesome cook so we had plenty of homemade donuts, cookies and bread all summer. My parents always had a beautiful vegetable garden which was a special treat for me. The whole family loved summer in Maine.

This particular summer while Nathan was still doing the enema routine, both of us were getting more and more frustrated. For the time and discomfort it caused him, I questioned whether it was even worth it. Apparently the doctor had success with some patients with this new procedure, but we weren't seeing it. Giving a child opium was another concern of mine. I really didn't feel comfortable even having it around.

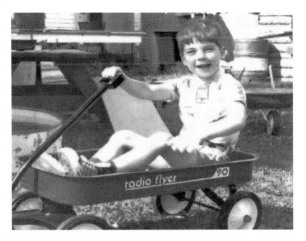

Finally, I had enough, and called the doctor who had put us on this program. I was nearly in tears, and she could hear the frustration in my voice.

"What do you want to do?" she asked.

"Quit! I want to quit!" I replied.

Her response ? "Go ahead."

"What?"

"Quit. Stop the enemas, but wean him off the opium," she replied.

I couldn't believe my ears! We could have quit at any time and yet we kept this struggle going for months because we didn't know there was a choice. At that point I didn't know if I should feel relieved or angry that she hadn't told me this before. I chose the former. Life is just too short to waste with anger. Now Nathan would be free and more relaxed to enjoy his summer, and I would, too.

One summer day Nathan was at his grandmother's round kitchen table with all of his cousins eating blueberry pie. My mother said, "Look at him," glancing toward Nathan. I looked his way but didn't notice anything except some pie on his face. She said it again, and I looked at all the kids around the table and noticed they were sitting on a chair but Nathan was standing beside his chair. When I looked again I noticed he was bleeding right through his shorts. My heart went to my throat and I gently went to him and led him out of the room to clean him up. The skin from the pull-thru surgery three years ago was still very sensitive. I was fighting back tears imagining how painful that must be for Nathan. He acted like everything was normal. It was hard for me to know how he was feeling because he seldom complained about pain - until he was a teenager. At that time he didn't like getting immunization shots. He could tolerate a lot of pain, just not shots.

Somehow I still didn't have the peace of mind I was looking for to send him off to kindergarten. One blessing of being on Governor's Island at this time was that there were choices for kindergarten. He could go a full day or a half day, so we chose the half day for Nathan. Since his birthday was September six, he was one of the youngest, just barely five, to start school. He still needed the afternoon rest.

Nathan had a very nice young teacher. His first day he came home all excited that his teacher looked just like Wonder Woman on TV. Hank decided he'd volunteer to go to the parent/teacher conferences! I think he agreed with Nathan.

He had to start kindergarten wearing a diaper until I was able to figure out a better way to keep him from getting soiled through his outer clothing. So far in our travels nobody was able to help with this dilemma. Eventually I remembered cutting the chux pads, disposable bed pads, to just the right shape to cover his colostomy when he was an infant. With some double sided tape, chux cut to the right shape to fit his underwear, and putting tape on the plastic side to hold in place, the problem was solved. Nathan would now be able to go without a diaper and not worry. I taught him how to discard his dirty ones, and he kept an extra in his jean pocket. I knew there would be obstacles for Nathan going to school.

We'd just have to trust God for that. Ultimately, I realized Nathan was God's child, on loan to us.

CHAPTER EIGHTEEN

PIANO LESSONS

The boys were doing well adjusting to a new baby in the house. Corey and Nathan shared the large bedroom and Paul had the small one. He would be going to kindergarten soon and I wanted him to get enough rest to be ready for school.

It seemed the right time for me to start giving piano lessons again. Since Charleston, when my first opportunity to get back into teaching piano was thwarted, because of our move , my heart had been longing for students once again. I put a card on the bulletin board in the lobby and a note in the classified section of the island paper, advertising piano lessons. Apparently there were few piano teachers on the island because within a few weeks a dozen students had signed up.

Since my teen years I'd been giving piano lessons off and on. The last couple of years at college I had a car on the campus and was able to give a few lessons then. After being married, having children, and moving so much there was no opportunity to have students until now. We felt this was the right time because we would be here for a few years, and with the cooperation of Hank and the boys I could get back to the thing I loved. Each student brought new challenges that I seemed to thrive on. So for a short time each day I wasn't just someone's wife or mother but once again, a piano teacher.

It had been four years since Nathan was born, and now he was doing so well he didn't need as much of my attention.

There actually was a little more time to run my fingers over the keyboard. The boys were very good playing together and also taking naps. Lessons were planned around naptimes and late afternoon after Hank got home from work. Paul and Nathan played upstairs in their rooms. There was a TV set in our bedroom if they needed to be quieted down. My piano students were never interrupted by rowdy kids. Corey was about five months old when I started teaching in New York, so if he wasn't napping Hank was holding him.

All of the piano students were at varying levels of accomplishment. One ten year old boy only wanted to play "The Entertainer". As much as we worked on new songs and exercises for technique, he would always come back playing only " The Entertainer!" That's probably why the parents sent him for lessons: to learn a new song. At first it was kind of comical but finally I had to tell him not to come any more. It was wasting his parents' money and my time. This young man definitely wasn't committed to learning anything new to play on the piano.

Another of my students wanted to pay me by crocheting a table cloth. That bought her lessons for a year, for her and her daughter. Unfortunately her daughter spilled a glass of chocolate milk on their piano keys, which ended lessons for both of them. Shortly after the accident on their piano, they received notice of a transfer off Governors Island. The mother had to finish my table cloth in a hurry so she could give it to me before they left. In her rushing she spilled coffee on this pure white cloth. But bleach took care of it nicely and I was more than pleased with the result. It turned out to be beautiful and a very special keepsake.

My best friend Pam, who lived next door, started taking piano lessons with me. I could hear her through the walls practicing for hours. We both had the same number of children and yet she found all that time to practice. I was so jealous! To my joy, I was actually forced to practice to keep up with her. She had taken lessons in her past and was a fast learner. Pam loved to try new things and would bring me music I'd never seen. So I had to keep ahead of her by putting in some extra practice time. The two of us had a lot of fun with the piano.

There was a particular student who became a very good friend of mine. He was a Captain in the Coast Guard who just loved music. Dick had enjoyed music his whole life and had played piano, as well as sang in choruses in his past. I always enjoyed the times he came and we often had coffee and a visit after the lessons. Dick and his wife enjoyed the opera and he liked to tell me about different ones they'd been to up in the city. Occasionally Dick would loan me a record or two. I didn't have much experience with opera, and it was fun to hear new and different music. The pleasure of talking to someone who loved music as I did made me realize how long I had suppressed that part of my life. Since Nathan was born, there was no occasion to teach or spend much time at all with the beautiful instrument that Hank bought me when we lived in Connecticut. However, now I loved spending time at the keyboard and stole a few extra minutes before and after the lessons. Something inside me started coming alive again; it was my love for making music. Much of this I owe to my good friend, Dick. He was an inspiration to me. The piano lessons continued until we got orders to leave New York.

Between Pam and Dick, I felt motivated to work on a recital again. This time it would be all music written by my piano teacher, John Dethier. Although he had passed away while we were living in Hawaii, this recital was important to me to honor his memory for his children, family, and friends. His music was unpublished, requiring the performer to read the original manuscripts. I spent hours one summer day in Blue Hill, going through old manuscripts at Mr. Dethier's son's house. Eventually I picked out just the right ones for a variety of his work. The concert consisted of music for two pianos, piano and voice, piano and cello, piano and violin, and some piano solos. There were a couple pieces for right hand alone, that he wrote when I was in high school. I had been studying a very difficult piece for left hand alone and asked Mr. Dethier if anyone had written for the right hand alone. He said he didn't think so. The very next week at my lesson he had two pieces newly written. The dedication on them was my name, which truly delighted me.

As time went on I became more and more determined that the recital be done the summer of 1981. It was scheduled for August in the Congregational Church in Blue Hill. I took a solid year to prepare for this and found my cellist and violinist at Kneisel Hall, a chamber music school in Blue Hill. My other pianist was Mary Cheney Gould, who directed and played for the Bagaduce Chorale. The vocal piece was done by Jackie Brownlow, the wife of the doctor who delivered Nathan. I felt almost driven to do this recital and didn't understand why until May 6, 1982, the day my Dad unexpectedly died. If I'd done the concert the following summer he would have missed it. In retrospect, it seemed the timing was for him; it pleased me to have done the concert when he could be there. He knew how hard I had worked for my piano lessons, and I knew the recital would mean a lot to him. The day of the recital Dad said to my mother, "Shouldn't we pass the hat or something?" We all laughed but I saw it as my Dad valuing all the hard work he knew I'd put into this recital.

The recital took place during our summer vacation in Maine. I spent as much time as possible at the keyboard, considering there were three little boys running around. Some days I actually had to find someone to watch them during my practice time, especially as the recital date approached. The recital was well attended and I was pleased Mr. Dethier's family was able to come. One of my strongest memories of that day was the end of the recital, during the applause, my oldest brother Sam, sitting in the front row, was the first to stand for me! That meant so much to me.

Dick had asked me, in the past, to join the choir in his church which was St. Patrick's in New York City. I had said no, because I was trying to get the boys into Sunday School at the Chapel on the island. To accomplish that would require consistency in attendance. I took them a few times, but they were still very young, and Hank wasn't very interested in helping me with that project. So after giving it a try we decided to wait until they were older.

Now the time came when I decided to audition for St. Patrick's Choir. Hank and I had talked about what it would mean if I was accepted. Rehearsals were Wednesday evenings and Sundays at 9a m, followed by the worship service. That would be extra time for him to be in charge of the kids alone. Hank agreed that he could handle things fine. So one Saturday afternoon Hank and I, pushing Corey in the stroller, took a walk up to St. Patrick's on Fifth Avenue where choir auditions were taking place. Hank took Corey for a walk around the area during this time. Dick happened to be there that day, helping with the auditions. I heard so many beautiful voices coming from that audition room before me that were rejected. It made me feel nervous that they'd never want me because my voice wasn't particularly strong. It turned out that was exactly what they were looking for. The director said he didn't need solo voices but the kind that would blend, especially altos. When I actually was accepted we were both surprised and excited; well, Hank was more surprised than excited! I honestly think he believed I'd never make it.

I had already asked Dick if I could go with him, because the subways and streets of New York were so unfamiliar to me. We arranged to meet at the ferry, the only way off the island. We'd run for the subway and then run for the church. It seemed everything in New York City was in a hurry. Sometimes if we got there a little early, we'd get coffee at a coffee shop right across the road from the church. When we got into the rehearsals, I saw quite a few other people had done the same thing. There were times during the rehearsal that the director would be explaining something in the music that Dick and I had discussed at a recent lesson. We both noticed these things, and would give each other a glance of acknowledgement.

St. Patrick's had a four manual pipe organ that was very massive and beautiful. The director was so talented he was able to direct us with one hand while accompanying us with the other, plus feet on the pedals. Occasionally he would bring in a few instruments to supplement the organ accompaniment. All together the choir of nearly 100, this huge pipe organ, plus extra instruments filled the church with a glorious sound. It was an unimaginable and unforgettable thrill of a lifetime to be in the midst of all that music! I will forever be grateful to my friend Dick for encouraging me to join the St. Patrick's Choir.

The whole experience of the choir was so elating for me. Surprisingly our processional hymns were usually ones I had learned growing up in the Baptist Church. Singing in this choir reminded me of my college choir. We even sang some of the same pieces, like various requiems and of course Handel's Messiah. I had never been in a Catholic Church before and felt the opportunity was a totally positive adventure.

CHAPTER NINETEEN

A MILITARY WIFE

I'd been in St. Patrick's Choir only a few months when Hank got orders that we were to go to Cape Cod. He would be on a ship, the *USCGC Unimak* , out of New Bedford, Massachusetts but we would be living at Otis Air Force Base in Bourne. We both were dreading the move, and Hank tried everything he could to stay in New York. Who would have thought? When we arrived in New York I was so unhappy, but now that we were leaving, once again my heart was breaking.

We left New York the week before Christmas, and the last Sunday at St. Patricks' we sang Handel's Hallelujah Chorus. It was such an awesome experience for me being in the midst of a choir of one hundred voices and singing that powerful song. It felt like this was the closest I'd get to Heaven in this life!

The last night we were in New York my friend Pam invited our family next door for dinner. We had a nice meal together, but the sadness Pam and I felt at never seeing each other again was overwhelming. Finally, she had to go to a class so she walked to the door, and without turning around, she said, "Good-bye, Sue," in a barely audible voice. Shocked that she'd say our last farewell in such a way, I responded, "Good-bye, Pam," and the door shut. I wanted to run after her and hug her and tell her we'd see each other again somehow. But I couldn't, and we wouldn't.

A military wife has no say in where she will live, how long she will be in that place, or when she will move again. That is unless she and her husband decide to buy their own home and leave the family in one place. In that case, she wouldn't see her husband very often. A wife goes where her husband is sent (if she can even do that). The husband is sent by directives from higher-ups who he doesn't know, and who have power over his and his family's life. We have little or no say in the direction our lives take. Nobody knows or cares that we've made new and dear friends, grown in new ways and experiences, and found security, joy, and love in new communities. No questions asked: it's time to go. It feels like the rug is being pulled out from under your feet.

Nathan knew that feeling when he was in high school. He was in junior high one year and high school three years in Cape May, New Jersey. He was comfortable, secure, and looking forward to graduating from Cape May Regional High School with his friends, when we got orders to move once more. He was so unhappy, and once again there was nothing that could be done to change the orders. Hank and I decided that if Nathan wanted to stay a year and graduate, he could, if he was able to find a friend to stay with. Meanwhile, the family was headed back to Maine. Hank was stationed in Boston but he decided he'd rather have the family in our own home in Maine, and come home whenever he was able to. We already planned to retire in Maine, so this would give the kids a little more stability. I was so happy when Nathan changed his mind and decided to come with us.

Sometimes life teaches us hard lessons. Looking back over the years, it's always easier to see why certain things happened as they did. An example for me is the Dethier Recital the summer before Dad died. It was so special to have him there and I know it meant as much to him as it did me. Also Nathan's high school graduation, which turned out to be in Blue Hill. There was a particular person that never would have been there had the graduation been anywhere else: my "angel next door," Carol. She had been living in Alaska and we hadn't seen her since the days when Nathan was an infant. She was visiting family in the area and was thrilled to be able to attend Nathan's graduation. It meant so much to her to finally see him grown and healthy.

As a military wife I learned to adjust to all the moving and inconveniences it brought. It was my job to make sure everyone was comfortable and happy in their new surroundings. It was my experience that, for the most part, the other wives were friendly and helpful. Military wives looked out for each other as neighbors. In 1978, we were living on Governor's Island and there was a terrible blizzard that stopped the ferry. It was impossible to come on the island or leave the island. Commissary and exchanges were closed, so we were very isolated. The storm continued for several days and then there was a knock on my door, and a lady, whom I did not know, passed me a bag containing baby bottle nipples. She said, "I thought there was a baby in this apartment and you might be able to use these." I thanked her and then realized my six-month-old baby was on his last nipple and I didn't have any spares! This incident felt like a hug or blessing from God. He does watch out for our needs even when we don't realize what they are.

Another time I was shopping at the commissary and had Corey, who was nearly a year old now, in a carriage. A lady came up to me, again a total stranger, and said, "That baby is too big for a carriage. I have a stroller I'm not using and we're moving. I'll give it to you." Once again I felt so undeservedly blessed.

In our travels I met many different military wives. Some of them made up their minds to hate their environment and dwell on the fact that they'd rather be somewhere else. They constantly complained about everything and seemed to make themselves and everyone around them miserable. Others just tolerated their new residence but their hearts and minds focused on where they'd been or were hoping to go next time. On the other hand, there were some wives who decided to make the best of wherever they lived. These wives looked for new opportunities and experiences for their families. They were the ones I learned from and decided I wanted to imitate. By taking chances to meet new friends and learn new skills, as well as visiting places I'd never been, my life was greatly enriched as a military wife.

There is a comradery among military wives, and while living in the allotted housing, many find strong friendships. Nearly everywhere we lived, I was able to find a particular friend to enjoy for the duration of living in that area. The kids were able to do the same thing; there were always plenty of children to play with in any military housing area. They all had something in common: their Dads worked for the government and were gone from the family often for long periods of time. Sometimes there were "duty days", which meant the service member would have to spend the night at work. For Hank, I remember one time that happened every six days. As he went up in rank he would have less duty days.

Wives would communicate, and the officer's wives would keep "enlisted wives" informed of when the ship, their husband was on, was coming home. Officer's wives would get together socially as a group, but in my experience the enlisted wives only did that if it was a gathering from a specific ship or duty station. There were very few times I was invited to join other wives socially because of my husband's duty station.

On Governor's Island there was a chapel that was used by both Protestants and Catholics. The Admiral's wife liked to invite all the wives from either of the church services to come for a special tea at her house. One other time the wives whose husbands were on the same ship had a get together. That was a mixture of officer and enlisted wives as well.

Hank did become an officer after many years in the service. He was an officer when we went to Cape May, our last duty station before moving home to Blue Hill. Hank's actual last duty station was Boston, where he spent ten years, before retiring, while the family lived in Maine.

CHAPTER TWENTY

CAPE COD

Living on Cape Cod we didn't see very much of Hank. He would be gone three or four weeks at a time, a couple of weeks in port, and then back out to sea again. I knew I had to be mom and dad for a while. The older boys had bikes, and there was a seat on the back of mine for Corey; he was only two and a half. Together the four of us biked all over the housing area. The terrain was mostly flat, with very few hills to make it difficult.

Once when Hank was out to sea the car wouldn't work. I was playing piano for Sunday morning services for the little chapel on base. So we rode our bikes to church and Sunday School, which wasn't too far for us. Some of the people in the church noticed we were without a vehicle and started showing up to fix my car. They were very thoughtful to do that, but I knew Hank would figure it out when he got home. The car wasn't very old and we'd never had trouble with it before, so I figured it probably wasn't too serious. It actually turned out to be a very small fuse in the dashboard that needed replacing. Meanwhile, if we all rode our bikes to the commissary we could get groceries that would fit in our baskets. Occasionally a neighbor would invite me to go shopping with her, so we were able to manage just fine.

Nathan had a wonderful second grade teacher at the school in the housing area. She displayed great compassion and caring towards the children. Often when I went to pick Nathan up after school she would have a child on her lap, making them feel so special. One day she talked to me about Nathan's condition and became very concerned. I had told her he should be allowed to go to the bathroom without asking because he couldn't control the bowel; extra clothing was in his back pack in case of accidents. She did some research and found a janitor's bathroom close to the classroom, where he could leave a change of clothes and use that bathroom. It seemed like a great idea and so I used it whenever he went to a new school, if circumstances would allow.

Memories of Cape Cod included meeting Hank's ship, the Unimac, covered in ice in January. The boys were holding signs we made saying, "Welcome Home, Dad!" as we stood freezing on the pier. Hank invited us on deck, which was covered with ice. The kids and I had to be very careful of our footing. It was a good opportunity for the boys to see where Dad worked, so we negotiated around the icy deck to get to his work station. This happened after he had been out to sea for a month or two.

We were only at Otis Air Force Base Housing for eighteen months. While Hank was deployed out to sea, and the boys in school, I needed to be doing something else. So I put my name into the Bourne schools to substitute. As a music teacher there were a lot of fun things I could do and call it "work". They wanted me to accompany a high school chorus as well as help individuals get ready for the All State try-outs. An accompanist for fourth grade violin classes was needed and that was particularly enjoyable. They also needed a teacher for some elementary music classes, and my favorite class that was called Special Ed. Those kids just loved to see me coming and would always try to do their best: a total delight to teach! I also was asked to put together a Christmas Program for one of the schools that turned out to be a lot of work, but rewarding, none the less. It's always fun to be paid for what you love doing.

Meanwhile, Corey was still very young, so we had to find a place for him. A military wife with whom I'd made friends, had a little boy and was willing to watch Corey as well. Her little boy was preschool, and he and Corey enjoyed playing together. One Easter, our husbands were out to sea so we had Easter dinner together at my house, the least I could do.

Nathan had a best friend when we lived on the Otis Base. He and Jesse would often walk to school together or with a group of kids from our area. Nathan remembers he was particularly impressed with his friend's drawing of cars. He had never seen anyone draw like Jesse. The boys were in second grade, and one day, walking home through the woods with a group of friends, one kid said, "Watch out for the females in the woods!" Nathan replied "What's a female?" The answer came back " They're monsters that live under rocks!" So Nathan and his friend, Jesse ran all the way home to avoid those monsters! You can imagine Nathan received a lot of teasing from his big brother when he got home.

Nathan told me another story about his kite that managed to get stuck in a tree just before going to Sunday school. He was so worried about the kite that he prayed that God would get his kite out of the tree. When he arrived home he was happy to find it had fallen onto the ground.

In the winter we got quite a lot of snow. Our quad-duplex was on a small hill which went down to a playground area, and we lived in the end unit. The houses were built around that playground so each house could see the children there, similar to Charleston. Hank built a ramp with snow. It gradually went from our backyard down the hill to the play area. All the kids in the neighborhood wanted to come slide on our hill and ramp. I was glad to see the kids happy near home. Hank also built a beautiful ramp of snow when we lived in Blue Hill. It went from our side yard to the back over the garden area. Now-a-days he builds ramps on the other side of the house for grandkids. After a storm he shovels all the snow off the deck in one place and that makes the high part of the ramp.

When we lived on Governor's Island there was a lady who lived about three doors down the hall from us, who was doing a Bible Club for kids. Figuring that I could get about one hour of rest, one afternoon a week, sounded good to me. Corey was still a newborn and keeping us up at night. The boys were invited, so after checking some of the basic beliefs she was teaching, I allowed them to go and was thankful for an hour of peace and quiet. They really enjoyed it and came home telling me stories each time. Here at the Otis Housing Area my mind went to finding another club like that for the boys, as I was feeling over-due for that peace and quiet! To find a place on Cape Cod to send the kids to this Bible Club, I wrote the lady in New York for suggestions. She answered with a seven page letter telling me exactly how to start this club. No! No! That wasn't what I meant! My plan was to send them, not teach them myself.

I'll never forget the day that letter came. The boys were playing while I was in the basement doing laundry, so I took the letter down to read it. Something came over me, and the tears welled up in my eyes; I didn't want to do this. Being mom and dad to three boys was exhausting for me and this was just one more thing. And for sure, Hank would not want to come home to find a bunch of kids in our house. So I started telling God all the reasons it couldn't be done in this home. But He wouldn't listen, and before even leaving the basement we were agreeing, if He would take care of Hank, I would do the club for the kids. When I went upstairs I felt myself going to get paper to write a poster announcing a "Good News Club" at my house at such and such a time. I was writing the date and time and didn't feel like it was me doing it. It was such a weird experience; nothing like that had ever happened to me before. The next day while the boys were in school, Corey and I took flyers to the homes around me and invited children we didn't even know to come.

On the designated date and time, my lesson plan prepared, fifteen kids showed up. We did songs, games, snacks, Bible stories and I even had an eighty- year -old man from the chapel on base that would come tell missionary stories. Mr. Livingston and his stories were my favorite part. Later, Nathan told me he felt the same. Mr. Livingston became a special friend of ours, and sometimes, when Hank was gone a long time, I'd have him over for dinner. Nathan and Paul loved hearing his true stories of missionaries in foreign lands. Mr. Livingston also told them on Sundays at the Chapel we attended. The club went on for eight or ten weeks and Hank was always working or out to sea. I'm not sure he ever knew we did this. God took care of His end and I tried to do mine. The communication I have with God is in my head, heart and scripture. It's often very clear to me what He expects from me.

When you're a military wife, you learn to "go with the flow". You look for opportunities that will make you and your family happy. Living that eighteen months at Otis Air Force Base was one of the hardest for me. 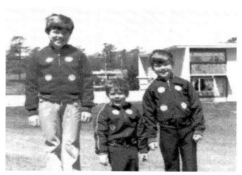 There were so many times when Hank was gone out to sea, which left me with the full responsibility of the three boys. It wasn't easy for him, either, since the seas were very rough in the northern waters in the winter. He had a problem with sea sickness more than when he was on other larger ships.

*   *   *

Hank became eligible to be sent to college by the Coast Guard for two years. He chose the University of Maine, as it was one of the colleges on the list for Electrical Engineering Technology . We lived in Blue Hill in our home, that we bought while living in New York. My parents were the brokers for the property, and my girlfriend's husband had built the house. We already knew the house; it happened to be the house where our wedding shower took place. My Dad had called us in New York, and we said we'd buy it the same day it went on sale. All the brokers in town said they never saw a house sell so fast!

From Otis Air Force Housing area, we headed north to Maine once again. This time it would be more than a summer vacation. The kids were excited to be living so close to their grandparents. Hank's daily commute to the University of Maine was just over an hour one way. We lived in our house for the first time, and of course he was eager to start making improvements. The house was a horrible shade of pink, and we couldn't wait to paint and work on it to make it our own. Therefore, when Hank wasn't in classes or working at the nearby Coast Guard Base, he was working on the house. Soon the putrid pink turned into a very pleasing shade of green. Many of the neighbors thanked us!

It was a very busy and taxing two years for Hank, dividing his time between his college courses, improvements on the house, and having any family time. Also, during this time we added a new member to our family, a little girl.

CHAPTER TWENTY-ONE

MAINE TO CONNECTICUT

Nathan was now in fourth grade, and Paul was in the fifth. Corey was still at home with me, still riding on the back of my bicycle. We liked to take rides downtown while the boys were in school. My parents' home was a little over a half mile from our house. My Dad had retired, and he was willing to watch Corey when I needed to go somewhere. Four-year- old Corey remembers having peanut butter sandwiches with Grampa. That was my father's staple for his life; almost every day he carried a peanut butter sandwich in his lunch pail. Corey had quite a few days with his Grampa, but not enough. Grampa passed away early in May, before Corey turned 5 at the end of that month. My Dad's passing left a huge hole in all of our lives; he died so unexpectedly.

Something very special needed to be done for Corey's birthday, so we gave him a kitten. I put it in a large box with a ribbon and let him open it. Corey called him Smurfy, because Smurfs were becoming popular on TV at the time. Smurfy was a bit of an unruly kitten, racing through the house and getting into everything. We all loved him and he was a good distraction for the family.

Nathan was a typical fourth grader. If you peeked into his classroom, you would not be able to pick him out as a child with any health problems. He was a Cub Scout and he liked to play baseball on the "Farm Team" in the summer, which was a town team, not school.

The two years we lived in our home the boys got to play with their cousins quite often. In the summer time Peter, Paul, Nathan, and Tobey would all go to day camp together. They loved hanging out and swimming, boating, and playing games all day together. It was a little hard for Nathan at times, but he learned how to take care of himself. At first I would get him after a half day, until he was comfortable staying a whole day. Corey and cousin Becky soon joined this crowd of campers, when they were old enough.

When Corey started kindergarten I decided to substitute in the schools. That kept me pretty busy, but still I was there when the boys got home in the afternoon. Corey was in first grade when we brought his new baby sister home. It had been a long time since we'd had the sounds of a newborn in the house! Emily was born in Blue Hill on November 1, 1983, just as Hank was finishing up at the University of Maine. He would be transferred to New London, Connecticut right after Christmas. Once again, he would be leaving me with a newborn, not to mention it was pretty hard for a dad to be away from his brand new baby girl! He lived in the barracks in New London until he could find housing appropriate for a family of six. We decided to let the kids finish the school year before moving the whole family. Now it felt like I was a single parent again. New London, Connecticut was about a seven-hour drive from us, so we didn't see Hank as often as we would have liked. Living near family made it so much easier than being across the country somewhere in another state. At this time my mother was just half a mile up the road, in a smaller house she'd built after selling the Parker Point house. She was more available if I needed her. She loved helping me with Emily, and being the grandmother of a little girl again.

Hank managed to come home for a long weekend about once a month. None of this was new to us but it did put a strain on family life. For example with him gone for several weeks at a time, I had some new rules that evolved, so when he came home, he was unaware of the changes. The boys would sometimes be disciplined for things I had allowed them to do or vice versa. It turned out to be very frustrating for all of us, but we did work through each situation as it came up. We called it "family growing pains."

At last there was a little girl in this family! In those days you couldn't find out in advance what gender the baby was. I felt numb for a couple days after giving birth, having been convinced we'd only ever have boys. Our friends and neighbors were so excited for us. News travels fast in a small town. My mother was flying pink ribbons on her car antenna, and we had pink booties taped to our picture window so everyone driving by knew it was a girl. Ours was a very happy household. All the boys wanted to hold their little sister, and Corey even wanted me to bring her for "Show & Tell" in first grade. The teacher and students were thrilled to see this beautiful little girl. It was such fun to have a baby in pink!

Esther Wood, a retired college professor and friend of ours from church, called me one morning before Emily was born. She said she'd had a dream that I had a girl and her name was Emily Jane Fenders, the most beautiful name she'd ever heard. Esther asked me to consider it and do what I wanted. So Hank and I talked and our daughter was born with that name on November 1, Esther's deceased mother's birthdate, which made it even more special for her.

After Emily was born, and Esther heard we'd chosen the name she suggested, she asked if she could be Emily's godmother. None of my children had a godparent so this was new to our family. Because Esther was so excited about Emily, we agreed. Esther wanted to take walks with Emily and me and she visited often, until we had to leave in the late spring when school was out. As Emily grew up we continued to visit Aunt Esther and have her over for meals with the family.

Nate & Emily

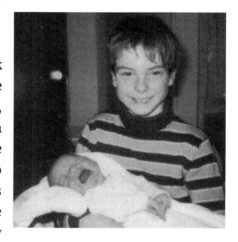

It was a long winter with Hank in Connecticut and the rest of the family in Maine. Reluctantly, Paul and Nathan helped me with the shoveling. In the house behind us lived a teenager who loved to drive the family's truck with a plow on it. He would come plow my driveway even when I hadn't asked him. It was a very thoughtful thing to do and the boys and I really appreciated the help on those stormy days.

During this time I was also fortunate to have a close friend, Ruth, who would come stay with my children one evening a week, while I attended a Bible Study with friends. It was especially generous of Ruth, since she had two small children of her own. She told me she enjoyed the children and liked reading to them, which they loved because we didn't always have time for a book at bedtime. It was great to have that evening to look forward to. Once again, God blessed me with a wonderful friend.

My Dad had passed away the year before Emily was born, so my mother was alone. She had decided to go back to work the day after my father's funeral, which I always considered an act of strength. My mother was a very strong person, and she had to deal with her sorrow in her own way. When she had some free time, she would try to help me by taking one of the boys for a while. That Christmas Corey was asking for a small Christmas tree for his bedroom, so Mom took him to find one. A shapely, small tree was found, and it fit nicely in Corey's bedroom. We located some Christmas decorations in the basement, just the right size for the tree. It accommodated his stuffed animals' Christmas in a very suitable way, and Corey seemed quite pleased with the whole situation in his room. Mom and Corey were both craving a little extra attention at a time when I really had my hands full. The Christmas tree search turned out to be just the "ticket" to fill that need.

By May I had started packing in preparation for the move to Connecticut. Hank was assigned a house that was very small and near a busy road. Because of his determination to get the right house that would fit our family, the housing department continued looking until they found one that was just right for us. Our new home would be a split level located in Ledyard. It had three bedrooms and a finished basement, with an attached garage. Eventually I put the three boys in the basement and they had plenty of room. It also had a huge back yard with an in-ground swimming pool. The owners had told us the pool wasn't working. However, Hank always liked fixing things, and that very first summer he had managed to get the pool working in short order. He kept it running in good condition the whole time we lived there.

It was a dream house for us, and we loved living in Ledyard. In the summer the kids were in the pool two or three times a day. When Hank got home from work, they'd all go in again while I made supper. It turned out to be an exceptional family activity for all of us together. I can't think of anything we all enjoyed as a family any more than that pool in the back yard!

We found so many good things about living in Ledyard, starting with the house and yard, which seemed to be designed for kids, our family specifically! Besides the pool in the backyard, there was lots of space for the kids to play. Shapely trees and bushes were placed around the house and large shade trees on the front and back lawns. The schools were some of the best in the country, so we were happy about that for the boys. We all agreed it was the best place for our family.

Stevie and Jim were wonderful next door neighbors. Stevie finally convinced me to go on walks after supper with her and her two dogs. We tried to walk every night, which was great exercise for both of us. Some hot summer nights we'd come back from a walk and jump in the pool for an evening swim.

Stevie invited us to her church, which was an Episcopal Church which later turned Anglican. I had never before attended this denomination, but the message was Biblical and the priest was so real in his preaching and his life, that we decided to try it. The kids attended Vacation Bible School and sometimes Sunday School.

When Emily was two, Hank got a call from a doctor that his sister Barb was in the hospital and he needed to come get his mother, with whom she lived. Virginia had muscle weakness in her legs and sometimes walked with a walker.

Her bedroom was upstairs in her house; she needed assistance using the stairs. Because of the urgency of the situation, Hank drove two hours home and surprised her. At first she didn't understand that Barb wouldn't be home, because the doctors had to hospitalize her when she went for her appointment. After Hank explained the situation to his mother, she agreed to come stay with us temporarily. Since her marriage, Virginia had always lived in her home in Newburyport, and the idea of leaving was very traumatic for her. Her husband had passed away a few years earlier, so she would have been completely alone. Hank convinced Virginia that this was the best for her and for Barb. Hank told his mom he would bring her back home when Barb was feeling better. We all went into this situation considering it to be temporary. None of us knew it would be for seven years, the rest of her life.

Virginia absolutely adored Emily. She loved to sit out on the porch and watch her playing. Emily amused her grandmother, who was more than entertained. The boys were running in and out of the back door to the back yard, and she enjoyed watching them too. Virginia relished watching the neighbor's bushes come into bloom one by one in the springtime. The porch wrapped around the side of the house, and Hank built a ramp in the back for her to use when she became wheelchair - bound. Virginia didn't want to sit in the sun too much so she stayed on the shady porch while I went up to the pool with the kids. We had a toddler wading pool near the big pool so Emily could play in that. It wasn't long before she was bored and ended up in the big pool. Emily was a vivacious child, always trying to keep up with three big brothers whom she adored, as they adored her! Whenever she was in the pool with the kids, she had some floating device on her and usually a brother right beside her, if I wasn't in there. Emily was too little to stand even on the shallowest end of the pool.

While we were in Ledyard, Hank became an officer in the Coast Guard. There was a special ceremony at the Coast Guard Academy in New London, where he was sworn in by the Admiral of the Coast Guard Academy. He went from Chief Petty Officer to Chief Warrant Officer, CWO. Our whole family, as well as some of the officials of the Academy, were present. My friend, Ruth, from Maine, and her complete family also came to witness this ceremony. We were all very proud of Hank, and decided to celebrate by going out to lunch at a very nice restaurant (the kind you normally wouldn't take kids). It was a special day for Virginia, particularly, to be able to see her son become an officer. She and I were both given corsages at the event.

Emily was also very fond of her grandmother, and would go in her room whenever she could. As she grew older she liked to lie on the foot of Virginia's bed and watch TV with her. We have a very sweet picture of them holding each other's hand. I was grateful my children could get to know their grandmother and have memories of her. It was obvious that their grandmother was happy to be with them also; the continuous activities of four children brightened her days. Emily grew up with Grammie Fenders in the house. Virginia passed away when Emily was just ten.

Emily &
Grammie Fenders

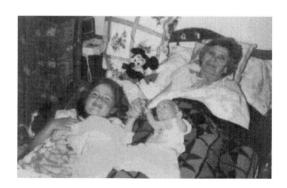

CHAPTER TWENTY-TWO

HEART SURGERY

Nathan did well as a fifth grader in the Ledyard school and with new friends. One day he came home and said, "Mom, I'm the last one to come in every time my class races in gym. Even the girls beat me!" I thought this was a little strange, but he had been having some therapy at school for his tight hamstrings, so I thought that might have something to do with it. Nathan wasn't the type of kid to whine and complain for no reason; he never did so from the time he was an infant. I think he was in second or third grade before I ever knew he had back pain all the time. Hank took him to a scoliosis specialist, who said he was borderline, and they wouldn't recommend doing anything at the time. We were told to keep an eye on it as he grew. This latest incident was a mystery.

One day the kids were in the pool, and I noticed Nathan didn't quite keep up with his brothers. Corey and Paul were swimming the length of the pool and diving off the deep end, while Nathan lingered in the shallow end with Emily. He loved playing with his little sister, so I didn't think much of it. I suggested that he swim the length of the pool for me, so I could watch him, but he said that he couldn't. After watching him try, it was obvious that he really wasn't able to. This became the second clue something was wrong. Hank and I decided not to wait for another one.

Hank took him to the doctors at the dispensary on base and they sent us to a cardiologist, who had replaced Dr. Whittemore, Nathan's cardiologist as an infant. He was very nice and recommended that Nathan go to Yale New Haven Hospital where he would do a Doppler Scan on his heart. This scan didn't give the cardiologist the information he needed. It showed there was a problem but it wasn't clear to the doctor, so the next step was for Nathan to have the heart catheterization. That was problematic for us because of our past experiences with that hospital. We had no good memories of that place. We both thought it would be better to go somewhere else, but the doctor told us if Nathan needed any surgery, the best pediatric cardiac surgeon in the country was located at that hospital. Hank and I agreed we wanted the best doctors for Nathan, so an appointment was made.

The day we took him we also brought Emily, while Paul and Corey stayed with their grandmother. It was a two hour ride for us to Yale New Haven Hospital. There were next-door neighbors who were our friends, and Virginia could call if she needed help. Everyone managed just fine. I'm not sure who took care of whom, the boys their grandmother or she them!

When we arrived at Yale New Haven they took us to the cardiac area and Nathan was put in a room. Next to his room was a playroom for children and family members. As we entered Nathan's hospital room and the nurse said the "fellow" would be right with us, my heart started pounding. I became very nervous and stressed because "fellow" was the title of a person we'd had before, when Nathan was five months old. I wasn't even sure what that title meant but knew I wanted a doctor. My mind went back to Dr. Bells' instruction to us: "Insist on seeing the doctor in charge." When she walked into the room and introduced herself I freaked! "Where's the doctor? I don't want a fellow, please call the doctor!" I was in such a state I had to leave the room and go into the playroom with Emily. Hank explained what we'd experienced at that hospital ten years ago when Nathan was an infant. How we didn't even recognize our child after ten days in the hospital, and how they did not take proper care of him. He told her that nothing was going to be done, this time, until we met the doctor doing the catheterization. The fellow and nurse were very kind and understanding and assured him many changes had been made, for the better, since those days. However, they did honor his wishes and we were able to talk to the doctor before the procedure. They were able to calm me down enough to win my confidence in this doctor.

During this whole emotional break-down of mine, Nathan was unaware of all we were talking about. He was in the playroom with his little sister while the discussion went on. As upset as I was, I couldn't let him be affected by my feelings just before going through this procedure.

Finally it was time for Nathan to get prepared for the catheterization. His father was present when the nurses came to give him a shot in the leg, and he didn't react at all. Hank said, "How come you let them give you a shot?" Normally he fought off anyone who came near him with a needle. Nathan's response was, " I couldn't say anything because the nurses were so pretty, I didn't want them to think I was a wimp!"

Nathan was allowed to choose any music he liked to be played during the catheterization because he would be conscious the whole time. The doctor told him he'd have to stay very still while they worked on him. They explained what was going to be done and how it would happen. The doctor forgot one thing: he failed to tell Nathan his head may get very hot. Nathan told me afterwards that his head started getting really hot, so hot it scared him and he started to panic. That's when the doctor got angry at him and told him if he moved at all they'd have to do the whole thing all over again! I guess that scared Nathan into tolerating whatever was happening in his head.

After the catheterization, we asked the doctor how Nathan did during the test. He said he did well, although was a little unruly. Later, Nathan confessed he was downright rude to the doctor. When his head was heating up and he felt like he was on fire, Nathan started swearing at the doctor, as he was trying to make him aware of his pain.

The catheterization showed Nathan had a hole in the top of his heart and was probably functioning with only one-third of his heart's capacity. The doctor who had done this catheterization suggested he be scheduled for surgery as soon as possible. We were told the pediatric surgical cardiologist that we wanted was overseas at this time and would be back in a few weeks. With that information, we immediately scheduled the surgery with him. Having heard such wonderful things about this surgeon, we wanted the best we could get for Nathan.

VACTERL association was a term we learned long after Nathan was born. The C does stand for cardiac problems but every child would not necessarily have the same heart problem. Just as everything else that happens to these children is not exactly the same. Over the years we've come to feel Nathan was one of the lucky ones, as each of his problems could have been much worse.

Nathans' teachers at school were very sympathetic and helpful. Knowing he would be out of school for a while, they arranged for a tutor to come to the house after the surgery. Surgery was scheduled for the early fall. My mother took a week off from her work to come stay with my family while Hank and I went with Nathan. It was a family event and everyone made concessions to help Nathan tolerate this ordeal.

Nathan was dreading the upcoming event, and I thought he might feel more support if we went to the Sunday night church service for prayer. The night before we took him to the hospital, I took him to church. The priest laid hands on him and prayed over him. It gave me more peace, and that's what was prayed for him: peace, healing, and pain control. When Nathan was put in a room after the surgery, the nurses kept coming in and offering him pain killers, but he always refused. He said he didn't need any, the pain was minimal. Both Nathan and I were so thankful that God heard our prayers.

Ruth, my friend from Blue Hill who stayed with the kids one night a week when Hank was away, was originally from that New Haven area. She had offered her parents' house if we needed a place to stay. Ruth was waiting at the hospital with her sister when we arrived. Her sister was a nurse at Yale-New Haven, and it was comforting to see them both.

Nathan was put on a ward with other pre-teens and teens. When the nurse hooked him up to the EKG machine, Nathan very calmly said "My heart's on the right side." She looked at us and said, "There's a comedian in every crowd," as she started to laugh. We said, "He's right." She tried again and found out he was right.

Nathan was quite upset and stressed out about the whole surgery that would take place the next morning. The nurse thought it would be a good idea if he saw where he would wake up when it was over. That seemed reasonable to me; I'd want to know. But Nathan was only eleven, and seeing patients in the intensive care recovery area with tubes in their bodies and hooked up to machines scared him, though he never said a word. I'm sure Nathan was thinking, "That's me tomorrow!" In retrospect, it wasn't a good idea for him. In hindsight (which is always 20/20), I felt bad that we had encouraged him to see that space with all the recuperating patients. It's so hard, as a parent, to know the right way to do these things.

We stayed with him through the evening and tried to help him get his mind off the surgery, but that was impossible to do. TV helped a little, but at that time there really weren't many evening programs that would interest kids. Without notice, Nathan had a real surprise! Ruth, our friend, came in with a special GI Joe Ninja toy that he had wanted. It was very hard to find, but she was persistent in her search because she knew how much he wanted this toy. She brought it in that night before surgery. It was a huge deal for him, and I was really happy he had something so meaningful to him that night. Nathan was allowed anything he wanted to eat, so he chose a large hot fudge sundae. These things made him relax a little, as he was dreading the following morning.

The next morning, breakfast was a sedative to keep him calm. The closer we came to surgery time, the more agitated and fearful he became. Finally it was time to put him on a gurney and take him to the cardiac surgery waiting area. None of us were prepared for what we would see, and it was obvious Nathan was terrified. Literally dozens of gurneys, it appeared, were lined up just waiting for their turn at surgery. This was the cardiac surgery area, so these were all heart patients. However the patients were not all children. Nathan took one look and went into a panic. We tried to calm him down, but the doctor had to give him another shot to relax him. That didn't even seem to help, and he was fighting the doctor and us, trying to get off the gurney. It was horrific for all of us! Finally the doctor had administered enough drugs to calm him down and we were told to leave. I felt like I was falling apart inside, myself. Nathan was really strong and just felt it necessary to fight, so the drugs didn't have the calming affect they should have. He recently told me that when they took him into the operating room, they asked him to count backwards from 100. Nathan remembers getting to 97 and falling asleep. Unexpectedly he woke up to the doctors and nurses talking, but he couldn't speak, so he kept blinking his eyes for someone to notice he was awake. When Nathan heard the doctor say, " Please pass the scalpel," he panicked and made himself go to sleep. We were told that the surgery would take about four hours and a nurse would come out to the waiting room with updates.

We waited for a while until a nurse came to tell us he was now in surgery and doing fine. She suggested we could go out for a walk or coffee or something, because it would be a while. So we went to a store and walked around, but neither of us could think of anything but getting back.

My friend Ruth and her sister were there waiting with us for quite a while. The hours passed, and I found myself pacing. We'd passed the four-hour mark long ago and nobody had given us a report. It was late and Ruth had to go home, so we were alone waiting. The hours ticked by and it was nearly nine hours; I was about to climb the walls! After checking the recovery room to see if they had forgotten to tell us he was back, I became concerned when the nurse said they had no news of Nathan. This information was more upsetting to me. Then I saw a man with a collar coming towards me, and my mind went crazy. He reminded me of my priest at the church we were attending.

He could see I was upset and right on the verge of falling apart. This stranger was so kind and gently came to me and asked, "Can I help?" I started to cry and told him I needed to see my son. He should have been out of surgery five hours ago and I'd heard nothing! At that moment, there was a gurney being wheeled down the hall and Nathan's surgeon was there. The doctor explained that he had found an extra artery that had to be clamped off. It was in a very precarious place and hard to reach, the reason why it took longer than expected. He said besides being on the wrong side, Nathan's heart was angled differently, which made it difficult to reach the area he needed to. The doctor also found that the hole in the top of Nathan's heart was larger than he had originally thought. The good news was everything went well, it just took extra time that the doctors hadn't expected.

Hank and I were so relieved--exhausted and relieved! They allowed us to see him after a while, but said he would sleep most of the night so we should do the same. That was the night I stayed with Ruth at her parent's house and she brought me back to the hospital early the next morning.

Meanwhile, Hank had to go home to take care of things there. His mother had decided to take to her bed. She wasn't sick or anything but she wanted to stay in her bed and have my mother wait on her. Hank went home to encourage her to try to cooperate with my mother, who was already taking care of two boys and a two year old. Virginia was in a wheel chair at the time, but was able to get around and take care of herself. It turned out Nathan was doing so well that Hank decided to stay home and help with things there.

When I went back to the hospital, I stayed in a large recliner chair beside Nathan's bed in the recovery area. He mostly watched cartoons on TV while he was in recovery. If he wasn't sleeping, the TV kept his mind off his body and any discomfort he might be feeling as the pain meds began to wear off. He couldn't talk for a while because of tubes, so I didn't try to talk to him much. Nathan remembers watching his favorite show, The Night Rider, when he closed his eyes, for what seemed like a few minutes but turned out to be four hours. When he woke up, he wanted to know what happened to his show.

The next day Nathan was able to go into a room, so he was placed in a room with an extra empty bed. The hospital allowed me to sleep in the other bed, as long as no patient needed it. There was a bathroom and shower and everything we needed there. He had food brought to him, and I went down to the cafeteria for meals, which was fine. Sleeping in a bed sure did beat a recliner! In the room, Nathan was hooked up to monitors that the nurses in the hall could watch. One time a suction cup came off and the machine flat-lined. Suddenly a flutter of activity was coming his way; alarms went off, and the nurses ran in to see if he was okay. It surprised him but he thought it was funny: all that clatter for nothing!

Nathan and I were there for about a week. Hank stayed home because I was able to be right with Nathan and he was doing very well. Soon he was up walking around and talking to people he met. Most of the time, Nathan slept, and when awake, spent his time watching TV. Hank was able to help my mother with the kids because she would soon have to go back to Maine. She had a job to get back to.

About five or six days after surgery Nathan was allowed to go home. We were both anxious to get back. Unfortunately, he came down with the flu just as we were making arrangements to leave. This delay was a huge disappointment to both of us.

However, it only meant one extra day in the hospital and then we were on our way. Nathan did real well healing but he was still out of school for a few weeks. The tutor came on a regular schedule, and Nathan was able to keep up with his classes. It was pretty boring for him just hanging around all day with Corey and Paul gone to school. His teacher and classmates had sent a plant and lots of get well cards and wishes. When it was time to go back to school, he was more than ready.

*   *   *

Nathan Remembers: school in Ledyard. He had been in the band in Blue Hill, but here they wouldn't let him join until he had some private lessons. That was a big disappointment for him because he really loved playing the trombone in the Blue Hill Band. He did get into the band in Ledyard, eventually, and until his high school graduation, he played in bands.

One day it was a storm day and the students were being dismissed early. It was also pizza day so they gave the kids their pizza and put them on the bus home. Nathan arrived home covered with pizza, and I was pretty upset about this. He still had his piece and couldn't understand why the other kids would want to throw theirs away in a pizza fight on the bus. It made no sense to me either. The mess on his coat was definitely not his fault.

The school was watching the Challenger Space Shuttle take off when it exploded. It left a horrific impression in the minds of those children, and Nathan still remembers it. We all thought it would be such a wonderful thing because they even had a school teacher on board. NASA had been very successful before and everyone expected success once again. Watching the event on TV was shocking and unpleasant for all who witnessed the explosion.

CHAPTER TWENTY- THREE

CAPE MAY

Nathan spent the rest of that school year recovering and getting stronger. By spring he had decided to join a group that were doing a walk-a-thon to raise money for the hungry. After checking with his doctor, he was pronounced fit for the task. This event turned out to be good for him, and although he was exhausted at the end, he enjoyed the activity.

We were all getting very comfortable living in Ledyard and not a bit happy when orders came in for another move. Hanks' mother, Virginia, didn't think she could go with us and wanted to move back with his sister. However, Barb had problems of her own and was no longer able to take care of her mother. With a lot of coaxing and encouragement, we assured Virginia it would be an adventure she wouldn't want to miss. Since she had no choice, other than a nursing home, she decided to try to make the best of the situation. Virginia had a big adjustment when she first came to live with us, and now there would be another uncomfortable move before her. I felt bad for her because she was elderly and had physical problems that exacerbated the whole ordeal for her. We were accustomed to the routine of moving every couple of years but this was all new to her.

In the spring, when the kids got out of school, we packed up and headed for Cape May, after spending two years in Ledyard, Connecticut. Now the moving van was loaded and on its' way with us not far behind. We had a Volkswagon van as well as a Volvo station wagon, so Hank drove one and I followed him in the other. He took the Volvo because it was easier for his mother to get in and out. She and Emily went with Hank, while I followed in the van with the three boys. We did well, considering drivers in Connecticut and New York do not like to leave space between themselves and the next car. Going at those fast speeds, I was uncomfortable being too close to the Volvo, so dropped back a car length or two, and someone would get right in front of me. Now we had the job of not losing sight of the rest of our family. Luckily the Volvo was orange and I had Paul in the front seat to help me keep track of it as we drove through the city of New York. In those days there were no cell phones. If we ever got separated I'd have been lost for sure. It all worked out and, although it was a stressful trip, we managed to arrive in Cape May at the same time. For later trips back and forth to Maine, we discovered other routes; our favorite used the Verrazano Bridge.

The new housing chosen for us was a huge disappointment. We'd definitely been spoiled by the beautiful house with the pool in Connecticut. In Cape May Housing, our home would be a duplex with four bedrooms. Each unit had a small enclosed backyard with a clothesline. Our front door faced a community playground, and once again we were at the end of a cull de sac, which is always a good thing with children. In military housing, you have to be inspected out of a place when you leave. If it's not perfect, you have to pay for someone to come clean after you leave. It was obvious to us that standards for different housing areas were not the same. After spending so much time and energy cleaning the house we left, Hank and I were crushed to see the work ahead, added to unpacking. Complaining never helps, so we got to work, which resulted in cleaning and unpacking at the same time.

Virginia was in the bedroom downstairs so she could easily get around in her wheel chair. Her room was right across from a full bathroom. There was a large bedroom upstairs we gave to the two oldest boys, and a very small room where we could put a bunk bed for nine-year-old Corey and Emily, three. Corey liked to listen to stories on the radio and read before he went to sleep, so we put him on the top. Emily slept on the bottom bunk where his flashlight didn't keep her awake. There was also a full bathroom upstairs as well as a master bedroom. These were cramped quarters for seven people, compared to what we came from. I was terribly displeased but learned to live with it. Other attributes of the housing area made up for the living quarters.

We were right outside the Coast Guard base where there was an awesome gym as well as an Olympic-sized swimming pool. There were also tennis courts we could play on at certain times of the day. The kids were very happy with all of this and I took them to the pool and gym many Saturdays.

Besides all that the base had to offer, there were basketball hoops between our buildings and the gate to the base. The hoops were placed in a big open field on a concrete pad. This field also provided plenty of room for the kids to fly kites. There were usually other kids around to play ball with and my boys spent a lot of time at that court.

While in Cape May, Corey was in a Cub Scout Troop; Hank and I were the den leaders. Every week we had seven or eight boys come to our house, and we'd help them with badges, learning knots, and many other things Scouts learn. One thing we did with them that wasn't to do with Scouts was their multiplication tables. The third grade class was learning them at this time and the boys liked to play a relay game before the Scout meeting began. So while we were waiting for everyone to arrive, we'd play a math game. The boys enjoyed it so much they would remind us if we forgot! To start the meeting, the boys would line up and say the Pledge of Allegiance and say all the Boy Scout Laws. Virginia loved these times and would come out of her room to watch them. Emily, now three, would line up beside the boys just as if she were one of them. Virginia got a kick out of her, and spent many hours watching and laughing at her antics. After spending time working on a badge, Hank would take them outside to run and play tag or other games, while I prepared the snacks.

On Corey's tenth birthday, he had a treasure hunt all around the area for his party. The treasure was a box full of candy that I gave to the guard at the base gate to hold for us. He turned out to be a good sport and played along. The boys had a lot of clues to follow before they ended up at the gate. That year May 29th was very hot in Cape May, which resulted in Corey's presents being mostly water guns of one sort or another. After the kids all soaked each other they continued to play outside until they dried off. Most of them lived in the housing area, and after the party they all walked home in damp clothes with lots of candy.

Emily's favorite thing to do was playing on the playground outside our door. I sometimes went over and visited with other mothers while the kids played. She was also visible from my kitchen window. Her best friend was a little boy named Matthew, who lived across from us. Each morning the two of them would run to greet each other with a big hug, and play on the playground for hours. Some days Virginia would sit outside in the sun and watch her play. She would laugh a lot at the things the kids would do. When the boys weren't playing basketball on the court or riding their bikes, they would be playing with remote control cars on the sidewalk in front of the apartment. The boys liked seeing their grandmother outside with them as Emily did. Virginia enjoyed meeting other neighbors and seemed to adjust well to Cape May. She soon learned to love the area and was disappointed when we had to leave.

While the boys were in school, I would often take Emily on the back of my bike and ride down to a nearby park or to the beach. The beaches seemed to go on forever. It was a truly beautiful spot in Cape May, where the water met the sky on the horizon and they were both a gorgeous shade of blue. Cape May had much to offer, with its' boardwalks and quaint shopping malls. Many specialty shops lined the streets, and you could find unique items that might not be found elsewhere. Our favorite was a 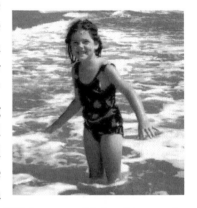 candle shop and, of course, Fudge Kitchen, which Grammie Fenders treated us to every year at Christmas and Easter.

The school Corey attended had a swimming pool, so their gym class was swimming lessons twice a week. He loved that; he also liked playing clarinet in the band. When he was in the sixth grade, he enjoyed playing basketball at school. It was a nice school and he had a lot of friends there. Corey and Nathan spent a lot of time on their bicycles in Cape May.

Nathan was in junior high school and seemed to be doing fine. And then he had a spell of being a "bear" every day when he came home. We couldn't figure out what was bothering him. His health issues seemed to be under control, and I kept asking if something was wrong, but got no response. It was unsettling to me because this was my even-tempered kid who now seemed to be turning into a monster at times. He'd come home from school and go directly to his room and shut the door. It surprised me, and we didn't know what to do, so we tried to give him as much space as possible. At this time one of the chores for the boys was doing dishes after supper. When it was their turn they had to wash and I would wipe. It turned out to be a good time for me to talk to them about their day. Even with the one-on-one with Nathan, I couldn't seem to make a break-through with his grumpiness.

Finally, there was an open house at school, so I went and visited all his classes and met all his teachers. The school was very large so there were a lot of teachers to visit. After meeting each teacher and introducing myself as Nathan's mom, I studied their faces. This is when I expected the moment of truth, when they'd tell me what was going on with him. No such luck; every one of them said what a wonderful person he was, so well behaved and polite. One teacher went so far as to say she wished she had more students just like him! To top it off, his academics were fine as well; now I was baffled. Apparently they didn't know any more than we did and Nathan wasn't sharing. So we figured it must be one of those growing stages kids go through. I suspected all kids react differently to this time in their lives and Nathan had a lot to deal with. It was a phase, and he did get through it and became his sweet, lovable self again.

Nathan recently told me while we were living in Cape May he was badgered and bullied by some kids on the basketball team. Nathan decided he wanted to play basketball, so joined the team. After about three practices, he realized this game just wasn't his thing. Nathan's theory was that the bullies on the team were so elated that he quit, consequently they totally ignored him thereafter. My theory is they saw him with his shirt off in the locker room, showing all the scars on his abdomen, and their consciences caused them to leave him alone. Although Nathan was disappointed to not participate in the sport, he had cleared a huge hurdle in his young teen life by facing the bullies!

Paul was in high school the whole four years we were in Cape May. His freshman year I visited the guidance counsellor to make sure he was adjusting into this new school. The campus was much larger than what he was used to, and Paul was always a little on the shy side when going to a new school. She was very nice and said she'd keep an eye out for him. One day Paul and I were talking about extra-curricular activities. He told me the school had a swim team that he'd like to join; but you have to have a physical and he didn't want that. So I called the school the next day and talked to my friend, the guidance counsellor, and she said, " The doctor is here today doing physicals and I'll send him right down." My mother−in−law thought I was terrible to do that, but he came home after school pretty happy that he's now on the swim team! He remained on the swim team for the full four years. Because his school didn't have a pool, some mornings he would leave as early as five a.m. to go to swim practice at another location with his teammates.

In the summer we still went to Maine for vacation. As the boys grew older they wanted jobs. One of Paul's first jobs was working for his Uncle Jon's construction business. The first thing he learned was how to dip shingles in stain for shingling houses. Later he was able to help with the addition on our house when we moved to Maine permanently. He and his cousin Peter worked together, and one summer Paul lived with their family most of the summer. Nathan had a job at a restaurant, called Uncle Bill's, on the beach at Cape May. The restaurant's specialty was pancakes and Nathan liked working there as a dishwasher, and everyone liked him as well. When it came time to go to Maine, he wanted to stay and work. He had a bicycle he could ride to work on, and Hank was there with him and his grandmother most of the summer. When Hank came to get us in Maine, his sister Barb came to stay with her mother and Nathan.

Nathan had a lot of good friends in Cape May. We attended a Methodist Church that had a large Youth Group that met a couple times a week. The church also had a gymnasium where the kids could have a game night every week. Paul was also part of the group. This became a large part of their social lives in high school. The group raised money every year by making and selling cookies and peanut brittle around Christmas time. The kids and parents would spend a Saturday in the church kitchen making the cookies and candy. It was an enjoyable day for all of us. Later the kids would take orders and deliver the food. They used the money for a ski trip in the Poconos during February vacation. It became a fun adventure for them to look forward to each year.

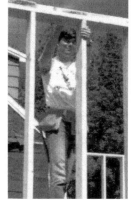

Virginia loved going for rides around Cape May, especially the boardwalk. Hank and I took the boys down on the boardwalk to a roller skating rink and left them for a while, as we took Emily and Grammie for a walk on the boardwalk - well, Grammie was riding the wheel chair, and Emily liked to push her. She loved candy and ice cream so the four of us found a place for a treat. There is a lighthouse near the end of the Cape, as well as a bird sanctuary that Virginia enjoyed. She thoroughly enjoyed the area, much more than she ever allowed herself to believe she would.

*   *   *

Cape May became the longest duty station time of Hank's career. After four years, even Virginia was feeling this was home and she was very unhappy to hear it was time to move again. When it came time to leave, nobody wanted to go, and once again there was no way to extend Hank's duty. He was being sent to Boston Coast Guard Base to be on another ship, the USCGC Escanaba, under strenuous objection of most of our family. Nathan especially wanted to finish his last year of high school in Cape May. He would be graduating from a different high school after attending only one year.

While we lived in Cape May I took a job as choir director at the Methodist Church we attended. The people in this choir were very dedicated and talented. Their former choir director had Parkinson's Disease and could no longer direct, but he could still sing, which made him a great encouragement to me and all the choir members. For almost two years, I had the privilege of directing this choir of thirty people. The church was large enough to have a good budget for music, which allowed me to buy any music I wanted. It was such a joy for me to work with these Christian people who loved to sing and praise God. The choir was made up of mostly seniors, who were very kind to me and my family.

The day we left Cape May was a Sunday afternoon after an Easter Service. The choir sang an arrangement of the Hallelujah Chorus in church that morning. As we were driving out of town, I turned the car radio on just in time to hear my choir singing. The service had been recorded and put on the radio that afternoon. Once again I was getting a send-off from a place I loved with the Hallelujah Chorus, while fighting back tears as we left.

Hank and I decided we didn't want to live in Boston, so this time we agreed the family would live in our own home in Blue Hill. Hank would be on the ship in Boston and come home whenever he could.

It was necessary to add another bedroom downstairs in our home for Virginia, so we spent the summer building an addition twenty-four feet by sixteen feet. It was a beautiful room with lots of windows for light. There were large glass doors on one end which in the future would open onto a deck. One end of the room was for Virginia's bed and the other was a sitting area for her to enjoy company. She dreaded leaving Cape May but, after she was settled in, Virginia managed to feel quite comfortable in Blue Hill. Upstairs was the same-sized room built for Paul and Nathan. The space was larger than any room they had ever shared before.

Hank tried to come home as many weekends as possible. It was about a six hour drive from our home to his duty station in Boston. At this point, Paul was at the University of Maine studying engineering and sharing a room with his cousin, Peter. Nathan was in his senior year at George Stevens Academy in Blue Hill, and not happy. He did know some of the kids because he was here for fourth and fifth grade. But he really liked Cape May and considered it home. Corey was in seventh grade in the Consolidated School and Emily was in first at the same. The year was 1990.

HIGH SCHOOL GRADUATION

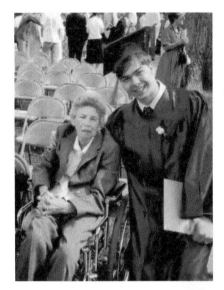

Nate & Grammie Fenders

Corey, Paul, Emily, & Nate

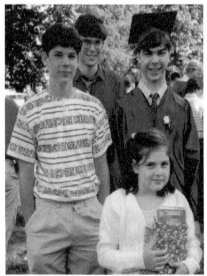

CHAPTER TWENTY- FOUR

NATHAN GOES TO COLLEGE

THE beautiful bedroom we built upstairs for Paul and Nathan was not used by them for very long. All their lives they had lived in small rooms they had to share, and now when we were in our own house and they finally had plenty of space, they were grown up and leaving home.

After Nathan's graduation he worked the summer at the local grocery store and went to Husson College in the fall. Paul was leaving for his sophomore year at the University of Maine at Orono. It felt like I'd lost two kids at once. I was happy they could go on with their lives without me, but at the same time many pangs of missing them.

At this point in Nathan's life his health issues were minimal and he was doing great. Nathan loved college and being independent. The only thing Husson lacked at the time Nathan was there was a college band. He had played in the band and jazz band at Stevens Academy his senior year. Nathan's instrument was his father's trombone. For his birthday I had bought him a trombone of his own, and now there was no band to play it in. He enjoyed living in the college dorm and was given a job as Resident Assistant on his floor. It was a job of responsibility, which happened to be one of Nathan's strong traits.

Near the end of Nathan's freshman year of college, he came home with his roommate one weekend. His roommate wanted me to know Nathan was struggling to breathe after walking up and down stairs or a distance to classes. Nathan was not a complainer and hadn't said anything to me about it. Immediately I insisted he visit our family doctor. He was feeling so badly that he couldn't object to my request. A blood test revealed his hemoglobin was down, and the doctor wanted to see him again. He continued to come home about once a week for several weeks and every time his hemoglobin would drop more. Our doctor could not find a place on Nathan's body where he was losing blood, and therefore saw no reason for the hemoglobin count to continue to decrease. Finally our family doctor scheduled a test in Bangor that was done on a large machine that he expected would give us the cause of his hemoglobin drop. Nathan and I were both feeling very weary of the run-around. Once again, we had no definitive answer about his condition.

We went for lunch after the test and had such a hopeless feeling. He wasn't doing any better, and our doctor seemed to feel this was the last resort for an answer. In retrospect, we found out the operator of the last test did not have the information about Nathan from his chart. He did not realize Nathan's internal organ placements were different than most, therefore he didn't scan the correct areas.

I had written a letter to Hank to explain the situation with Nathan. He was out to sea and had to use the MARS system (ham radio operators) to call me to discuss what to do for Nathan. At the end of each sentence we had to say "over." We decided to make arrangements to take him to Boston for an evaluation. I called Children's Hospital and they had us bring him right down. Within three hours the doctors found a Meckels Diverticulum. This was a congenital growth caused by blood slowly dripping into a pouch off the side of his colon. Over time it had grown to nearly the size of an orange. As soon as they discovered this he was scheduled for surgery.

The whole ordeal was extremely hard on Nathan. I simply will say Dr. Lund, that did this surgery, recognized his own handwriting on Nathan's records from his infanthood. He had been an intern during Nathan's earlier surgeries with Dr. Eraklis. Nineteen years later he was still helping people in the same department we took Nathan as a baby.

Dr. Lund did a great job. Nathan went on to have one more less complicated surgery the following year, and has done well ever since. All together Nathan had twelve surgeries, nine were before the age of two.

*   *   *

Nathan met his wife-to-be, the second year of college. Nancy was a freshman at Husson College. Like his dad, he knew right away that she was "the one". He brought her home for us to meet, and the second time he brought her home Nancy had something to show us. After we'd had dinner together and they were nearly ready to leave, she showed us a diamond ring on her finger. I was speechless to say the least! I honestly thought my heart would stop beating. How long had they known each other? Could they really decide so quickly to get married? We hardly knew her, but they were so happy and young! We congratulated them and talked for a while and they left.

When they left, the tears started to flow and I had flashbacks of Nathan being two, sitting on the floor at our first house in Connecticut. At the time I was doing the dishes after supper and was so frustrated he wouldn't eat anything. He toddled into the kitchen and sat on the floor. I put some left over cold carrots, cauliflower, and broccoli in a plastic dish and passed it to him without saying a word, never dreaming he'd eat them. He surprised me and ate all of them!

And today he told me he's getting married! My Nathan was now her Nathan and I was dissolved in tears. Somehow I would pull myself together and be happy that he was so happy.

Life throws you those curve balls every once in a while. You try so hard to raise your children the best way possible and take care of all their physical, spiritual, mental, and emotional needs. Suddenly, unexpectedly, they say, "I'm getting married." And you wonder where did the years go? From that point on, they were together in another world, and we didn't see him nearly as much as we wanted to, although, that did change substantially when the children came along.

Following Nathan's graduation from college they got married. He was twenty two and she was twenty. He had a job working for MBNA for the first couple years of their marriage while Nancy finished school. MBNA closed down and left many people out of jobs but Nathan was always able to find something. Nancy, graduated two years later, and then went for her Masters. She is now a Registrar at a local college and he works an IT job for a health care facility. They have two beautiful children, a son, Jonathan and a daughter, Dakota, and a very busy, happy life together. At this writing, they have been married for twenty-two years.

Nathan is a devoted husband and dad and continues to show his strong personality traits of honesty, integrity, faithfulness, and a great sense of humor. He loves the Lord, and is true to his beliefs. Nathan has a strong moral fiber and teaches his children well. He is civic-minded and has spent time being a Scout Leader as well as an Assistant Leader. Nathan is still easy-going and slow to anger. Life was never easy for him; there have always been hard times physically, as well as the expected challenges of raising children. I'm very proud of who he is and how he handles life situations as they come along. I believe his experiences as a child gave him the strength and fortitude to handle the rough times of life. As we all must agree, life is hard: it's how you handle it that determines who you are.

*   *   *

A recent quote from Nathan that surprised me, showing his character, seems appropriate to put here. He said, "Mom, if I had the choice to go back and have my life different, I don't think I would change anything. The way I was born and all I went through made me who I am today. It also made you and Dad who you are today." He is so right about that in so many ways. We learned our priorities had to change when a child is born with many health issues. When things became difficult for us, as parents we had to consider the child's needs before our own. Plans we'd made for our lives had to be second place to the medical needs of Nathan. Because of Nathan's birth problems, Hank stayed in the service not the six years he planned, but a total of thirty years. There was never a consideration for Hank getting out of the service until we knew Nathan's health needs were taken care of completely. If Hank had left the service after six years, we probably would have come back to Blue Hill. He would have gone to the University of Maine for a degree in education and become a math teacher. He always had that goal in the back of his mind because he loved math and taught it to all of our kids.

Our lives would all have been very different. The kids would have missed out on the travelling opportunities we experienced throughout their growing up years. We never would have known the many friends we made in all the places we were stationed.

More importantly, how would Nathan's life have been changed? Maybe he would have had a whole different outlook on life. We'll never know exactly how much of his personality might have been affected by the challenges of his early life. Years later, would he have chosen to have lunch with the popular guys, calling after him, on the first day at a new school? Or would he still be the kind of person who'd go by them and sit with the kid nobody else would sit with? Would he have been the kind of teenager that needed the same kind of sneakers his friends had? Would he have been more interested and demanding of material things to match his peers? We'll never know and I kind of liked what we got. Nathan has always been a humble person who cares about other people and especially the downcast. Only God in His infinite wisdom knows what the outcome of Nathan's life could have been, had he been born without VACTERL association. As for me, I'll take what we got and be thankful for all the wonderful gifts God gave us all wrapped up in Nathan.

In conclusion, I would like to say how blessed I've been to have married the man I did and have the family we had together. Every one of our children has been a challenge and a joy all in one. Nathan had the health issues and I call it a privilege to be his Mom. He has always been a blessing to us and our family.

I am thankful to God for always being there for us. One of my life verses has been, "Trust in the Lord with all your heart and lean not to your own understanding. In all of your ways acknowledge Him and He will direct your path." Proverbs 3: 5 and 6. So much of raising Nathan had nothing to do with "my understanding," because his health issues were way beyond my understanding. But I do acknowledge Him in His love and mercy He has blessed me and my family in a million ways! God has always directed us into the right path to find answers to our confusion and inadequacy. My other life verse, "I can do all things through Christ who strengthens me." Philippians 4: 13. When times were hard and I felt so weak, I knew there was a loving God who cared even for the little problems in life. There were times, like the first time we saw Nathan after his first surgery, when my mind screamed, "I can't!" That verse got me through then, and through a lot of hard days to follow.

This book would not have been written without the support of my Heavenly Father. He gave me encouragement in so many ways and through many friends and relatives. But more than that, He helped me with memories I had tucked away in my mind for years. Many mornings I would wake up with a whole chapter in my mind. He gave me all the titles; they were so automatic for me. And He gave me better ways of saying things that I'd already written. He's been with me throughout this whole project and He's been with me throughout my whole life!

My prayer is that this book will give encouragement to the hurting population of people who feel alone, especially those with VACTERL association and their care-givers. When life gets difficult we sometimes want to throw up our hands and quit! It's perseverance fueled with love that keeps us going through the tough times. Love held our family together when there seemed to be no answers and no place to turn. My hope is that this book will help more people to understand the struggles the VACTERL association population has every day of their lives.

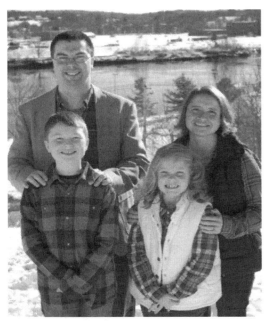

FAMILY PICTURE: NATHAN, NANCY, JONATHAN, and DAKOTA

ACKNOWLEDGEMENTS

I would like to acknowledge the support of my family and friends during this long project. Especially my husband Hank, whom I depended upon for pictures and computer help. I am thankful for my friend, Julie Nicholson who was a great encouragement throughout this writing. Also Nancy Hodermarsky and Nancy Werth who helped me with the editing of early chapters. My four children all helped in various ways either with technical problems or memories of their youth. Thank you all !

Made in the USA
Middletown, DE
11 March 2019